Qigong Wisdom

Ancient Practices for Modern Life

Mei Lin Zhang

Xspurts.com

A New Zealand Designed Product

Other Versions Available

Why limit yourself to just one format?

This book is now available in physical, digital, and audiobook options.

Choose the way you love to read and dive into the story today. You won't regret it!

Digital ISBN: 9781776968237
Physical ISBN: 9781776968220
Audio ISBN:

To obtain a different format of this book at a discounted price, please get in touch with us at:

http://isbn.xspurts.com/

Contents

Have Questions / Comments?

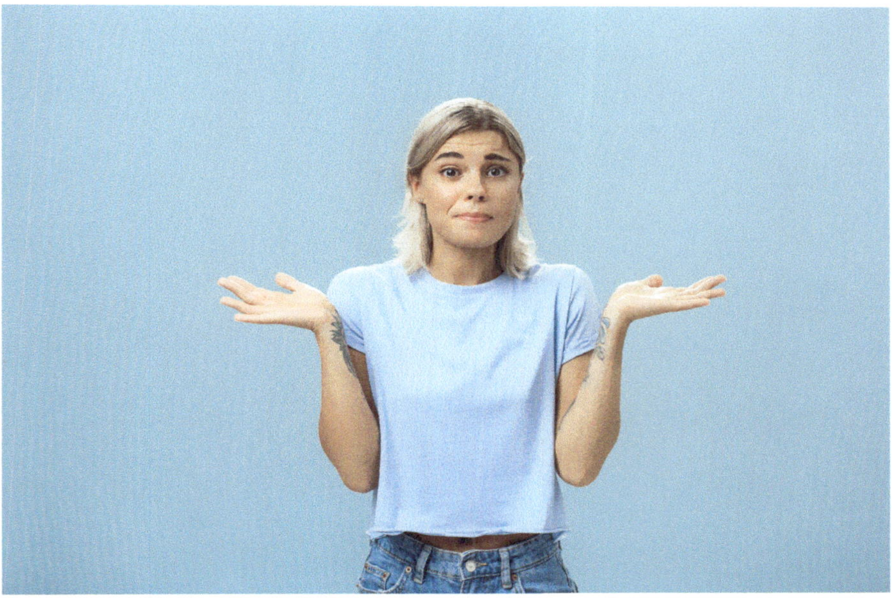

This book was designed to cover as much information as possible, but I know I have probably missed something, or some new amazing discovery has just come out.

If you notice something missing or have a question that I failed to answer, please get in touch and let me know. If I can, I will email you an answer and also update the book so others can also benefit from it.

Thanks For Being Awesome :)

Submit Your Questions / Comments At:

https://questions.xspurts.com

Get Free Stuff

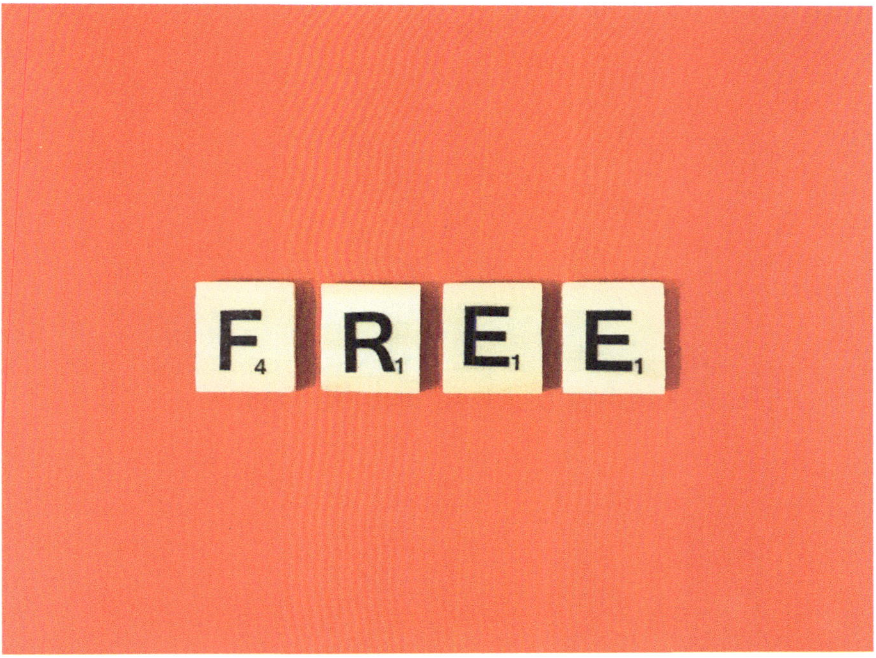

We love writing and have produced a huge number of books.

For being one of our amazing readers, we would love to offer you more books we have created, 100% free.

To claim this limited time special offer, simply go to the site below and enter your name and email address.

You will then receive loads (as we love our readers so much :) of our great books, content and audio direct to your email account, 100% free!

Get Loads of FREE Stuff at:

https://free.xspurts.com

Chapter One

Introduction to Qigong

Qigong, pronounced as "chee-gong," is an ancient Chinese practice that has been around for thousands of years. The word Qigong can be broken down into two parts: "Qi," which refers to the life force energy that flows within us, and "Gong," which means to work or cultivate. Therefore, Qigong translates to "cultivating life force energy."

Qigong is a holistic practice that focuses on the coordination of breath, movement, and meditation. It is often referred to as a "moving meditation" because it involves slow, flowing movements that are synchronized with deep breathing techniques. Qigong is believed to help balance the flow of Qi throughout the body, which in turn can lead to improved health and wellbeing.

There are many different forms of Qigong, each with its own unique set of movements and breathing techniques. Some styles are more focused on martial arts, while others are more geared towards health and wellness. Some common styles of Qigong include Tai Chi Qigong, Medical Qigong, and Daoist Qigong.

Tai Chi Qigong is one of the most popular styles of Qigong and is often practiced for its health benefits. It involves slow, graceful movements that are performed in a continuous sequence. Tai Chi Qigong is known for its ability to improve balance, flexibility, and coordination, as well as reduce stress and anxiety.

Medical Qigong, on the other hand, is a form of Qigong that is used for therapeutic purposes. It involves a trained practitioner using various Qigong techniques to help restore balance and harmony to the body. Medical Qigong is often used to treat chronic pain, stress-related disorders, and other health conditions.

Daoist Qigong is a form of Qigong that is rooted in Daoist philosophy and focuses on cultivating the body's inner energy to achieve a state of harmony and balance. It involves various postures, breathing techniques, and meditation practices that are designed to activate the body's natural healing abilities.

One of the key principles of Qigong is the concept of Qi. Qi is believed to be the vital life force energy that flows throughout the body and is responsible for maintaining health and wellbeing. According to traditional Chinese medicine, when Qi is flowing smoothly throughout the body, we experience good health and vitality. However, when the flow of Qi becomes disrupted or blocked, it can lead to various health problems.

Qigong is believed to help balance the flow of Qi throughout the body, which can improve health and wellbeing. By practicing Qigong regularly, we can strengthen the body's energy system, reduce stress and anxiety, and improve overall physical and mental health.

In addition to its physical and mental health benefits, Qigong is also a spiritual practice for many people. It is often used as a way to connect with the divine and cultivate a deeper sense of inner peace and harmony. Qigong is also a way to connect with nature and the natural rhythms of the universe.

History and Philosophy of Qigong

Qigong, an ancient Chinese practice that involves the coordination of breath, movement, and meditation, has a rich history and philosophy that is deeply rooted in traditional Chinese culture. The history of Qigong dates back over 5,000 years, with the first references to Qigong appearing in ancient Chinese texts such as the Huangdi Neijing (The Yellow Emperor's Classic of Internal Medicine) and the Dao De Jing (The Book of the Way and Its Power).

According to legend, Qigong was first developed by a legendary Chinese emperor named Huang Di, who is credited with writing the Huangdi Neijing. The book contains descriptions of various Qigong practices, including breathing exercises, meditation techniques, and movements that are designed to promote health and longevity.

Over the centuries, Qigong has evolved and developed into many different styles and forms. In the 1950s, the Chinese government began to standardize Qigong practices and created a system of Qigong exercises that could be taught to the general public. This led to a widespread interest in Qigong throughout China, and eventually, it began to spread to other parts of the world.

The philosophy of Qigong is deeply rooted in traditional Chinese culture and is based on the principles of Taoism, Buddhism, and Confucianism. One of the key principles of Qigong is the concept of Qi, which is believed to be the vital life force energy that flows throughout the body. Qi is believed to be responsible for maintaining health and wellbeing, and when it is flowing smoothly throughout the body, we experience good health and vitality.

Another key principle of Qigong is the concept of Yin and Yang, which are opposing forces that are believed to exist in all things. Yin represents the passive, feminine, and receptive aspects of nature, while Yang represents the active, masculine, and assertive aspects of nature. According to Qigong philosophy, health and wellbeing are achieved when Yin and Yang are balanced and in harmony.

The practice of Qigong is designed to help balance the flow of Qi throughout the body and promote harmony between Yin and Yang. Qigong involves various movements, breathing techniques, and meditation practices that are designed to activate the body's natural healing abilities and promote overall health and wellbeing.

There are many different styles of Qigong, each with its own unique set of movements and breathing techniques. Some styles are more focused on martial arts, while others are more geared towards health and wellness. Some common styles of Qigong include Tai Chi Qigong, Medical Qigong, and Daoist Qigong.

Tai Chi Qigong is one of the most popular styles of Qigong and is often practiced for its health benefits. It involves slow, graceful movements that are performed in a continuous sequence. Tai Chi Qigong is known for its ability to improve balance, flexibility, and coordination, as well as reduce stress and anxiety.

Medical Qigong, on the other hand, is a form of Qigong that is used for therapeutic purposes. It involves a trained practitioner using various Qigong techniques to help restore balance and harmony to the body. Medical Qigong is often used to treat chronic pain, stress-related disorders, and other health conditions.

Daoist Qigong is a form of Qigong that is rooted in Daoist philosophy and focuses on cultivating the body's inner energy to achieve a state of harmony and balance. It involves various postures, breathing techniques, and meditation practices that are designed to activate the body's natural healing abilities.

In addition to its physical and mental health benefits, Qigong is also a spiritual practice for many people. It is often used as a way to connect with the divine and cultivate a deeper sense of inner peace and harmony. Q

The Health Benefits of Qigong Practice

Qigong is an ancient Chinese practice that involves the coordination of breath, movement, and meditation. It is a holistic practice that has been found to have numerous health benefits. Here are some of the health benefits of Qigong practice:

1. Reduces stress and anxiety: One of the primary benefits of Qigong practice is that it can help reduce stress and anxiety. The slow, flowing movements of Qigong, combined with deep breathing techniques, can help calm the mind and promote relaxation. This can lead to a reduction in stress and anxiety levels, as well as an improvement in overall mental wellbeing.

2. Improves balance and coordination: Qigong involves slow, controlled movements that require a great deal of balance and coordination. Regular practice of Qigong can help improve balance and coordination, which can be especially beneficial for older adults who may be at risk for falls.

3. Boosts the immune system: Qigong has been found to have a positive impact on the immune system. Regular practice of Qigong has been shown to increase the number of white blood cells in the body, which are responsible for fighting off infections and diseases.

4. Reduces chronic pain: Qigong has been found to be effective in reducing chronic pain, such as back pain, arthritis, and fibromyalgia. The slow, gentle movements of Qigong can help increase circulation and reduce inflammation, which can alleviate pain and discomfort.

5. Improves cardiovascular health: Qigong has been found to have a positive impact on cardiovascular health. Regular practice of Qigong has been shown to reduce blood pressure, lower cholesterol levels, and improve overall cardiovascular function.

6. Enhances mental clarity and focus: Qigong can also improve mental clarity and focus. The deep breathing techniques used in Qigong practice can help oxygenate the brain, which can improve cognitive function and enhance mental clarity.

7. Improves flexibility and range of motion: Qigong involves slow, controlled movements that can help improve flexibility and range of motion. This can be especially beneficial for individuals with conditions such as arthritis, which can cause stiffness and limited mobility.

8. Promotes better sleep: Qigong practice has been found to promote better sleep. The relaxation and stress-reducing benefits of Qigong can help improve the quality of sleep, leading to increased energy and improved overall health and wellbeing.

9. Supports digestive health: Qigong has been found to have a positive impact on digestive health. Regular practice of Qigong has been shown to improve digestion and alleviate symptoms of digestive disorders such as irritable bowel syndrome (IBS).

10. Enhances overall health and wellbeing: Perhaps the most significant benefit of Qigong practice is its ability to enhance overall health and wellbeing. Regular practice of Qigong can help improve physical, mental, and emotional health, leading to a greater sense of wellbeing and vitality.

The Connection Between Qigong and Traditional Chinese Medicine

Qigong is an ancient Chinese practice that involves the coordination of breath, movement, and meditation. It is a holistic practice that is deeply rooted in traditional Chinese culture, and is closely tied to traditional Chinese medicine (TCM). In fact, Qigong is often considered to be a form of TCM, and is often used in conjunction with other TCM practices such as acupuncture and herbal medicine. Here is a closer look at the connection between Qigong and traditional Chinese medicine:

The philosophy of TCM is based on the concept of Qi, which is believed to be the vital life force energy that flows throughout the body. Qi is believed to be responsible for maintaining health and wellbeing, and when it is flowing smoothly throughout the body, we experience good health and vitality.

Qigong is designed to help balance the flow of Qi throughout the body, which can promote health and wellbeing. Qigong involves various movements, breathing techniques, and meditation practices that are designed to activate the body's natural healing abilities and promote overall health and wellbeing.

Many of the movements and postures used in Qigong are based on the principles of TCM. For example, some Qigong postures are designed to stimulate specific acupuncture points on the body, which can help regulate the flow of Qi and promote healing.

In addition to its physical health benefits, Qigong is also used in TCM as a way to promote emotional and mental wellbeing. Qigong is often used to treat conditions such as anxiety, depression, and insomnia, which are believed to be caused by imbalances in the flow of Qi.

In TCM, the body is seen as a complex system of interconnected parts, and any health problem is believed to be the result of an imbalance or disruption in the flow of Qi. TCM practitioners use various techniques, including acupuncture, herbal medicine, and Qigong, to restore balance and harmony to the body.

Qigong is often used in conjunction with other TCM practices to help promote overall health and wellbeing. For example, a TCM practitioner may recommend Qigong exercises to be done in conjunction with acupuncture or herbal medicine treatments.

Medical Qigong is a specific form of Qigong that is used for therapeutic purposes. It involves a trained practitioner using various Qigong techniques to help restore balance and harmony to the body. Medical Qigong is often used to treat chronic pain, stress-related disorders, and other health conditions.

Medical Qigong practitioners are trained in TCM theory and practice, and use Qigong techniques to treat specific health conditions. For example, a Medical Qigong practitioner may use Qigong exercises to help improve circulation, reduce inflammation, and alleviate pain.

Chapter Two

Understanding Qi and Qigong

Qigong is an ancient Chinese practice that involves the coordination of breath, movement, and meditation. At the core of Qigong practice is the concept of Qi, which is the vital life force energy that flows throughout the body. Understanding Qi and how it relates to Qigong is essential for anyone who wants to fully appreciate and benefit from this ancient practice.

Qi is a fundamental concept in traditional Chinese culture, and is believed to be the vital life force energy that flows throughout the body. According to traditional Chinese medicine, Qi is responsible for maintaining health and wellbeing, and when it is flowing smoothly throughout the body, we experience good health and vitality.

There are different types of Qi in the body, including Yuan Qi, which is the prenatal Qi that we inherit from our parents, and Zong Qi, which is the Qi that is produced by the lungs and used to power the body's vital organs.

One of the key principles of Qigong is to balance the flow of Qi throughout the body. Qigong involves various movements, breathing techniques, and meditation practices that are designed to activate the body's natural healing abilities and promote overall health and wellbeing.

The movements used in Qigong are designed to stimulate the flow of Qi in the body. By moving the body in a slow, flowing manner, Qigong practitioners can help improve the circulation of Qi throughout the body, leading to improved health and vitality.

The breathing techniques used in Qigong are also designed to promote the flow of Qi in the body. Deep breathing techniques, such as abdominal breathing and reverse breathing, can help activate the body's natural healing abilities and promote relaxation and calm.

Meditation is another key component of Qigong practice. Through meditation, Qigong practitioners can focus their minds and cultivate a sense of inner peace and harmony. This can help reduce stress and anxiety, and promote overall mental and emotional wellbeing.

There are many different styles of Qigong, each with its own unique set of movements and breathing techniques. Some styles are more focused on martial arts, while others are more geared towards health and wellness. Some common styles of Qigong include Tai Chi Qigong, Medical Qigong, and Daoist Qigong.

Tai Chi Qigong is one of the most popular styles of Qigong and is often practiced for its health benefits. It involves slow, graceful movements that are performed in a continuous sequence. Tai Chi Qigong is known for its ability to improve balance, flexibility, and coordination, as well as reduce stress and anxiety.

Medical Qigong, on the other hand, is a form of Qigong that is used for therapeutic purposes. It involves a trained practitioner using various Qigong techniques to help restore balance and harmony to the body. Medical Qigong is often used to treat chronic pain, stress-related disorders, and other health conditions.

Daoist Qigong is a form of Qigong that is rooted in Daoist philosophy and focuses on cultivating the body's inner energy to achieve a state of harmony and balance. It involves various postures, breathing techniques, and meditation practices that are designed to activate the body's natural healing abilities.

The Concept of Qi

Qi is a fundamental concept in traditional Chinese culture, and is at the core of practices such as acupuncture, herbal medicine, and Qigong. Understanding the concept of Qi is essential for anyone who wants to fully appreciate and benefit from these ancient practices.

The concept of Qi is complex, and has many different meanings depending on the context in which it is used. In general, Qi is the vital life force energy that flows throughout the body, and is responsible for maintaining health and wellbeing.

According to traditional Chinese medicine, Qi is believed to flow through a network of channels, or meridians, throughout the body. When the flow of Qi is smooth and unobstructed, we experience good health and vitality. However, when the flow of Qi is disrupted or blocked, we may experience symptoms of illness or disease.

There are different types of Qi in the body, including Yuan Qi, which is the prenatal Qi that we inherit from our parents, and Zong Qi, which is the Qi that is produced by the lungs and used to power the body's vital organs.

One of the key principles of Qigong is to balance the flow of Qi throughout the body. Qigong involves various movements, breathing techniques, and meditation practices that are designed to activate the body's natural healing abilities and promote overall health and wellbeing.

The movements used in Qigong are designed to stimulate the flow of Qi in the body. By moving the body in a slow, flowing manner, Qigong practitioners can help improve the circulation of Qi throughout the body, leading to improved health and vitality.

The breathing techniques used in Qigong are also designed to promote the flow of Qi in the body. Deep breathing techniques, such as abdominal breathing and reverse breathing, can help activate the body's natural healing abilities and promote relaxation and calm.

Meditation is another key component of Qigong practice. Through meditation, Qigong practitioners can focus their minds and cultivate a sense of inner peace and harmony. This can help reduce stress and anxiety, and promote overall mental and emotional wellbeing.

In addition to its role in traditional Chinese medicine and Qigong, the concept of Qi has also been explored by modern science. While the existence of Qi as a tangible, measurable substance has not been proven, modern research has found that practices such as Qigong and acupuncture can have a positive impact on the body's physiological systems, including the nervous system, immune system, and cardiovascular system.

The Three Dantian Energy Centers

In traditional Chinese medicine and Qigong practice, the body is seen as a complex system of interconnected parts, and the flow of Qi is believed to be essential for good health and wellbeing. The Three Dantian Energy Centers are key points in the body where Qi is believed to be stored and circulated. Understanding the Three Dantian Energy Centers is essential for anyone who wants to fully appreciate and benefit from Qigong practice.

The Three Dantian Energy Centers are located along the body's central energy channel, or the Ren Mai channel, which runs from the perineum to the crown of the head. Each Dantian is associated with a specific type of Qi and is responsible for a different aspect of physical, mental, and emotional wellbeing.

The Lower Dantian is located in the lower abdomen, approximately two inches below the navel. It is also known as the "Sea of Qi," and is the primary storage center for Qi in the body. The Lower Dantian is associated with the body's physical energy and vitality, and is responsible for maintaining the health and wellbeing of the organs in the lower abdomen, such as the kidneys, bladder, and reproductive organs.

The Middle Dantian is located in the center of the chest, at the level of the heart. It is also known as the "Sea of Spirit," and is the primary storage center for the body's emotional and mental energy. The Middle Dantian is associated with the emotions, intuition, and creativity, and is responsible for maintaining the health and wellbeing of the heart and lungs.

The Upper Dantian is located at the center of the forehead, between the eyebrows. It is also known as the "Sea of Wisdom," and is the primary storage center for spiritual energy. The Upper Dantian is associated with the intellect, intuition, and higher consciousness, and is responsible for maintaining the health and wellbeing of the brain and nervous system.

Each Dantian is associated with a specific type of Qi, or energy, and can be activated and balanced through Qigong practice. Qigong exercises are designed to stimulate the flow of Qi in the body and activate the Three Dantian Energy Centers. By practicing Qigong, we can help balance the flow of Qi throughout the body, leading to improved health and vitality.

Some common Qigong exercises that are designed to activate the Three Dantian Energy Centers include:

1. Lower Dantian Breathing: This exercise involves focusing on the breath and directing it to the Lower Dantian. By breathing deeply into the lower abdomen, we can stimulate the flow of Qi and activate the body's physical energy and vitality.

2. Middle Dantian Meditation: This exercise involves focusing on the emotions and directing them to the Middle Dantian. By cultivating a sense of inner peace and calm, we can activate the body's emotional and mental energy and promote overall wellbeing.

3. Upper Dantian Visualization: This exercise involves visualizing a bright light at the center of the forehead, and directing the breath to the Upper Dantian. By focusing on the intellect and higher consciousness, we can activate the body's spiritual energy and promote a sense of inner wisdom and insight.

Yin and Yang in Qigong

In traditional Chinese philosophy, Yin and Yang are two complementary principles that represent the balance and harmony of the universe. In Qigong practice, the principles of Yin and Yang are used to describe the flow of energy in the body, and are essential for understanding and practicing Qigong effectively.

Yin and Yang are often described as opposite and complementary forces that exist in a state of dynamic balance. Yin represents the feminine, passive, and receptive aspects of the universe, while Yang represents the masculine, active, and assertive aspects. Together, Yin and Yang represent the duality of existence and the natural balance of the universe.

In Qigong practice, the principles of Yin and Yang are used to describe the flow of energy in the body. According to traditional Chinese medicine, the body is made up of two types of energy, Yin energy and Yang energy. Yin energy is associated with the body's internal organs, such as the liver, kidneys, and heart. Yang energy is associated with the body's external organs, such as the muscles, bones, and skin.

In order for the body to be healthy and balanced, the flow of Yin and Yang energy must be balanced and harmonious. When the flow of Yin and Yang energy is disrupted or imbalanced, we may experience symptoms of illness or disease.

Qigong practice is designed to balance the flow of Yin and Yang energy in the body, and promote overall health and wellbeing. By practicing Qigong exercises that are designed to activate and balance the body's Yin and Yang energy, we can promote a sense of inner balance and harmony.

Some common Qigong exercises that are designed to balance the body's Yin and Yang energy include:

1. Tai Chi Qigong: This exercise involves slow, flowing movements that are designed to activate the body's Yin and Yang energy. Tai Chi Qigong is known for its ability to improve balance, flexibility, and coordination, as well as reduce stress and anxiety.

2. Yin Qigong: This exercise involves slow, gentle movements that are designed to activate the body's Yin energy. Yin Qigong is often used to promote relaxation and calm, and is known for its ability to reduce stress and anxiety.

3. Yang Qigong: This exercise involves more vigorous movements that are designed to activate the body's Yang energy. Yang Qigong is often used to increase energy and vitality, and is known for its ability to improve overall physical fitness.

In addition to its role in promoting physical health and wellbeing, the principles of Yin and Yang are also essential for understanding and practicing Qigong meditation. Qigong meditation involves focusing the mind and cultivating a sense of inner peace and harmony. By focusing on the principles of Yin and Yang, we can cultivate a sense of inner balance and harmony, and promote overall mental and emotional wellbeing.

Chapter Three

Basic Principles of Qigong Practice

Qigong is an ancient Chinese practice that combines physical movements, breathing techniques, and meditation to cultivate and balance the body's energy, or Qi. Qigong has been practiced for thousands of years, and is known for its ability to promote overall health and wellbeing. Understanding the basic principles of Qigong practice is essential for anyone who wants to fully appreciate and benefit from this ancient practice.

Relaxation

One of the key principles of Qigong practice is relaxation. Qigong exercises are designed to be slow, gentle, and relaxing, with the aim of calming the mind and body. By relaxing the body, we can help reduce stress and tension, and promote a sense of inner peace and calm.

Breathing

Another key principle of Qigong practice is deep breathing. Qigong exercises are designed to be synchronized with the breath, with the aim of promoting deep, slow breathing that can help calm the mind and improve circulation. By focusing on the breath, we can activate the body's natural healing abilities, and promote overall health and wellbeing.

Posture

Good posture is essential for effective Qigong practice. Qigong exercises are designed to be performed with an upright, relaxed posture, with the aim of improving balance, alignment, and overall physical wellbeing. By maintaining good posture during Qigong practice, we can help improve circulation, reduce tension, and promote overall health and wellbeing.

Mindfulness

Mindfulness is an essential component of Qigong practice. Qigong exercises are designed to be performed with a focused, present-moment awareness, with the aim of cultivating a sense of inner peace and calm. By practicing mindfulness during Qigong, we can reduce stress and anxiety, and promote overall mental and emotional wellbeing.

Movement

Movement is a fundamental aspect of Qigong practice. Qigong exercises are designed to be slow, gentle, and flowing, with the aim of promoting overall physical fitness and wellbeing. By practicing Qigong movements, we can improve flexibility, coordination, and overall physical fitness, leading to improved health and wellbeing.

Visualization

Visualization is another key aspect of Qigong practice. Qigong exercises often involve visualizing the flow of Qi through the body, with the aim of promoting overall health and wellbeing. By visualizing the flow of Qi through the body, we can activate the body's natural healing abilities, and promote overall health and wellbeing.

Posture and Alignment

Posture and alignment are essential components of effective Qigong practice. Qigong exercises are designed to be performed with an upright, relaxed posture, with the aim of improving balance, alignment, and overall physical wellbeing. Understanding the importance of posture and alignment is essential for anyone who wants to fully appreciate and benefit from Qigong practice.

Good posture is essential for effective Qigong practice. Qigong exercises are designed to be performed with an upright, relaxed posture, with the aim of improving balance, alignment, and overall physical wellbeing. By maintaining good posture during Qigong practice, we can help improve circulation, reduce tension, and promote overall health and wellbeing.

Poor posture, on the other hand, can lead to a variety of physical problems, including back pain, neck pain, and headaches. Poor posture can also affect our mental and emotional wellbeing, leading to feelings of stress and anxiety.

When practicing Qigong, it is important to maintain good alignment throughout the body. Alignment refers to the positioning of the body's bones and joints, and is essential for proper movement and function. Good alignment helps to distribute the body's weight evenly, reducing strain on the muscles and joints.

Proper alignment begins with the feet. The feet should be shoulder-width apart, with the toes pointing straight ahead. The weight of the body should be evenly distributed between both feet.

The knees should be slightly bent, with the hips slightly tucked under. This helps to maintain a neutral pelvis and protect the lower back.

The spine should be straight, with the shoulders relaxed and the chest open. The head should be held upright, with the chin slightly tucked in.

When performing Qigong movements, it is important to maintain good alignment throughout the body. This helps to ensure that the movements are performed safely and effectively, and can help to prevent injury.

In addition to its physical benefits, good posture and alignment can also have a positive impact on our mental and emotional wellbeing. By maintaining good posture and alignment, we can cultivate a sense of inner strength and confidence, leading to improved self-esteem and overall mental and emotional wellbeing.

Some common Qigong exercises that are designed to improve posture and alignment include:

1. Standing Meditation: This exercise involves standing in a relaxed, upright posture, with the aim of improving balance, alignment, and overall physical wellbeing.

2. Wuji Standing: This exercise involves standing in a neutral, relaxed posture, with the aim of promoting relaxation, calm, and balance.

3. Spinal Twisting: This exercise involves twisting the spine gently from side to side, with the aim of improving spinal mobility and promoting overall physical wellbeing.

Breathing Techniques

Breathing techniques are an essential component of Qigong practice. Qigong exercises are designed to be synchronized with the breath, with the aim of promoting deep, slow breathing that can help calm the mind and improve circulation. Understanding the importance of proper breathing techniques is essential for anyone who wants to fully appreciate and benefit from Qigong practice.

Breathing is a fundamental aspect of life, and proper breathing techniques are essential for overall health and wellbeing. Breathing affects many aspects of our physical, mental, and emotional health, including our heart rate, blood pressure, and stress levels.

In Qigong practice, breathing is used to cultivate and balance the body's energy, or Qi. Qigong exercises are designed to be synchronized with the breath, with the aim of promoting deep, slow breathing that can help calm the mind and improve circulation.

Proper breathing techniques in Qigong involve breathing deeply and slowly, using the diaphragm and abdominal muscles to control the breath. This type of breathing is known as abdominal breathing, or diaphragmatic breathing.

Abdominal breathing involves breathing in deeply through the nose, filling the lungs with air, and expanding the belly outward. The breath is then held briefly, before exhaling slowly through the mouth, allowing the belly to contract inward.

Abdominal breathing is essential for effective Qigong practice, as it helps to promote deep relaxation and calm, while also improving circulation and promoting overall health and wellbeing.

Some common Qigong breathing exercises include:

1. Abdominal Breathing: This exercise involves focusing on the breath, and using the diaphragm and abdominal muscles to control the breath. Abdominal breathing is essential for effective Qigong practice, and can help promote deep relaxation and calm.

2. Reverse Breathing: This exercise involves breathing in through the mouth, while pulling the belly inward. This type of breathing is used to promote the flow of energy in the body, and is often used in more advanced Qigong practice.

3. Counted Breathing: This exercise involves counting the breath, with the aim of promoting focus and concentration. By counting the breath,

we can bring our attention to the present moment, and cultivate a sense of inner calm and balance.

In addition to its physical benefits, proper breathing techniques can also have a positive impact on our mental and emotional wellbeing. By practicing deep, slow breathing, we can reduce stress and anxiety, and promote a sense of inner peace and calm.

Meditation and Mental Focus

Meditation and mental focus are essential components of Qigong practice. Qigong exercises are designed to be performed with a focused, present-moment awareness, with the aim of cultivating a sense of inner peace and calm. Understanding the importance of meditation and mental focus is essential for anyone who wants to fully appreciate and benefit from Qigong practice.

Meditation is an ancient practice that has been used for thousands of years to promote mental and emotional wellbeing. In Qigong practice, meditation is used to cultivate a sense of inner peace and calm, while also promoting mental and emotional clarity.

There are many different types of meditation, but they all involve focusing the mind on a particular object or idea, with the aim of cultivating a sense of inner calm and balance.

In Qigong practice, meditation is often combined with physical movements and breathing techniques, creating a holistic practice that promotes overall health and wellbeing.

Mental focus is also essential for effective Qigong practice. Qigong exercises are designed to be performed with a focused, present-moment awareness, with the aim of promoting mental clarity and focus.

By practicing mental focus during Qigong, we can improve our ability to concentrate, and cultivate a sense of inner calm and balance.

Some common Qigong meditation and mental focus exercises include:

1. Standing Meditation: This exercise involves standing in a relaxed, upright posture, with the aim of promoting mental and emotional clarity, as well as physical balance and alignment.

2. Mindful Breathing: This exercise involves focusing on the breath, and using the breath as a tool for cultivating inner peace and calm.

3. Visualization: This exercise involves visualizing the flow of Qi through the body, with the aim of promoting overall health and wellbeing.

In addition to its mental and emotional benefits, meditation and mental focus can also have a positive impact on our physical health. By promoting relaxation and reducing stress and anxiety, meditation can help to lower blood pressure and improve cardiovascular health.

Chapter Four

Qigong Warm-Up Exercises

Qigong warm-up exercises are an essential component of effective Qigong practice. These exercises are designed to prepare the body and mind for the physical and mental demands of Qigong practice, while also promoting overall physical fitness and wellbeing. Understanding the importance of Qigong warm-up exercises is essential for anyone who wants to fully appreciate and benefit from Qigong practice.

Qigong warm-up exercises often involve gentle stretching, breathing, and movement, with the aim of promoting circulation, improving flexibility and coordination, and reducing tension and stress.

Some common Qigong warm-up exercises include:

1. Joint Rotations: This exercise involves gently rotating the joints of the body, with the aim of improving flexibility and mobility, and promoting circulation.

2. Neck Stretches: This exercise involves gently stretching the muscles of the neck, with the aim of reducing tension and promoting relaxation.

3. Shoulder Shrugs: This exercise involves shrugging the shoulders up and down, with the aim of promoting relaxation and reducing tension in the shoulders and neck.

4. Arm Swings: This exercise involves swinging the arms gently back and forth, with the aim of promoting circulation and improving flexibility in the shoulders and arms.

5. Leg Swings: This exercise involves swinging the legs gently back and forth, with the aim of promoting circulation and improving flexibility in the hips and legs.

In addition to these warm-up exercises, Qigong also often incorporates breathing techniques and mindfulness exercises, helping to promote relaxation and focus, and preparing the mind and body for the demands of Qigong practice.

By practicing Qigong warm-up exercises regularly, we can improve our physical fitness and wellbeing, reduce stress and tension, and promote overall health and vitality. Whether you are interested in Tai Chi Qigong, Medical Qigong, or Daoist Qigong, there is a style of Qigong that can benefit you. With regular practice, Qigong can help promote overall health and wellbeing, leading to a happier, healthier life.

Joint Loosening Exercises

Joint loosening exercises are an essential component of Qigong practice. These exercises are designed to promote mobility, flexibility, and circulation, while also reducing tension and promoting relaxation. Understanding the importance of joint loosening exercises is essential for anyone who wants to fully appreciate and benefit from Qigong practice.

As we age, our joints can become stiff and less mobile, leading to a variety of physical problems, including pain and discomfort. Joint loosening exercises are designed to counteract these effects, promoting mobility and flexibility in the joints, and reducing the risk of injury and discomfort.

Qigong joint loosening exercises often involve gentle, repetitive movements that target specific joints and muscle groups, with the aim of promoting circulation and improving range of motion.

Some common Qigong joint loosening exercises include:

1. Ankle Circles: This exercise involves gently rotating the ankles in a circular motion, with the aim of promoting mobility and flexibility in the ankles.

2. Knee Bends: This exercise involves bending the knees slightly, with the aim of promoting circulation and flexibility in the knees.

3. Hip Circles: This exercise involves gently rotating the hips in a circular motion, with the aim of promoting mobility and flexibility in the hips.

4. Shoulder Rolls: This exercise involves rolling the shoulders forward and backward, with the aim of promoting mobility and flexibility in the shoulders.

5. Wrist Circles: This exercise involves rotating the wrists in a circular motion, with the aim of promoting flexibility and mobility in the wrists.

By practicing joint loosening exercises regularly, we can improve our physical fitness and wellbeing, reduce stress and tension, and promote overall health and vitality. These exercises can also be particularly beneficial for those with joint pain or stiffness, helping to reduce discomfort and promote healing.

In addition to joint loosening exercises, Qigong also incorporates breathing techniques and mindfulness exercises, helping to promote relaxation and focus, and preparing the mind and body for the demands of Qigong practice.

Stretching and Flexibility

Stretching and flexibility are important components of Qigong practice. These exercises are designed to promote mobility and flexibility, while also reducing tension and promoting relaxation. Understanding the importance of stretching and flexibility is essential for anyone who wants to fully appreciate and benefit from Qigong practice.

Stretching is the process of lengthening the muscles and tendons, with the aim of promoting mobility and flexibility. Regular stretching can help to improve range of motion, reduce the risk of injury, and promote overall physical fitness and wellbeing.

In Qigong practice, stretching is often combined with breathing techniques and mindfulness exercises, creating a holistic practice that promotes overall health and wellbeing.

Some common Qigong stretching exercises include:

1. Forward Bend: This exercise involves bending forward at the waist, with the aim of stretching the muscles of the back and legs, and promoting relaxation and stress reduction.

2. Chest Stretch: This exercise involves standing with the arms extended behind the back, with the aim of stretching the muscles of the chest and shoulders, and promoting improved posture.

3. Hamstring Stretch: This exercise involves sitting with the legs extended forward, and reaching forward to touch the toes, with the aim of stretching the muscles of the legs and improving flexibility.

4. Butterfly Stretch: This exercise involves sitting with the soles of the feet together, and gently pushing the knees toward the ground, with the aim of stretching the muscles of the inner thighs and hips.

In addition to stretching exercises, Qigong also incorporates joint loosening exercises, breathing techniques, and mindfulness exercises, helping to promote relaxation and focus, and preparing the mind and body for the demands of Qigong practice.

By practicing stretching exercises regularly, we can improve our physical fitness and wellbeing, reduce stress and tension, and promote overall health and vitality. These exercises can also be particularly beneficial for those with joint pain or stiffness, helping to reduce discomfort and promote healing.

Activating Energy Circulation

Activating energy circulation is a key component of Qigong practice. This involves promoting the flow of Qi, or life force energy, throughout the body, with the aim of promoting overall health and wellbeing. Understanding the importance of energy circulation is essential for anyone who wants to fully appreciate and benefit from Qigong practice.

Qi is believed to flow through the body along channels known as meridians. When the flow of Qi is blocked or disrupted, it can lead to a variety of physical and emotional problems, including pain, illness, and stress.

Qigong exercises are designed to activate and promote the flow of Qi, helping to improve overall health and wellbeing. By practicing Qigong regularly, we can improve our ability to circulate Qi, promoting physical and emotional balance and harmony.

Some common Qigong exercises for activating energy circulation include:

1. Meridian Tracing: This exercise involves tracing the meridians of the body with the fingertips, with the aim of promoting circulation and improving overall health and wellbeing.

2. Qi Ball: This exercise involves visualizing a ball of energy in the hands, and moving it through the body along the meridians, with the aim of promoting the flow of Qi and improving overall health and wellbeing.

3. Sound Healing: This exercise involves using specific sounds to activate the flow of Qi along the meridians, with the aim of promoting physical and emotional balance and harmony.

In addition to these exercises, Qigong also incorporates breathing techniques and mindfulness exercises, helping to promote relaxation and focus, and preparing the mind and body for the demands of Qigong practice.

By practicing exercises for activating energy circulation regularly, we can improve our physical fitness and wellbeing, reduce stress and tension, and promote overall health and vitality. These exercises can also be particularly beneficial for those with chronic pain or illness, helping to promote healing and improve overall quality of life.

Chapter Five

Qigong Forms and Techniques

Qigong forms and techniques are an important aspect of Qigong practice. These forms and techniques are designed to promote the flow of Qi, or life force energy, throughout the body, and to promote overall health and wellbeing. Understanding the different Qigong forms and techniques is essential for anyone who wants to fully appreciate and benefit from Qigong practice.

Qigong forms refer to the specific movements and postures that are used in Qigong practice. These forms can vary depending on the style of Qigong being practiced, but generally involve gentle, flowing movements that promote circulation, flexibility, and relaxation.

Some common Qigong forms include:

1. Eight Brocades: This is a popular Qigong form that involves eight different movements, each designed to promote the flow of Qi through a different meridian of the body.

2. Five Animals: This is another popular Qigong form that involves movements inspired by the movements of five different animals - the tiger, deer, bear, monkey, and crane.

3. Tai Chi: This is a popular Qigong form that involves a series of flowing movements that are performed slowly and gracefully, with the aim of promoting circulation, flexibility, and relaxation.

Qigong techniques refer to the specific practices and exercises that are used in Qigong practice. These techniques can vary depending on the style of Qigong being practiced, but generally involve breathing, visualization, and mindfulness exercises.

Some common Qigong techniques include:

4. Deep Breathing: This technique involves taking slow, deep breaths, with the aim of promoting relaxation and reducing stress.

5. Meditation: This technique involves focusing the mind on a specific object or idea, with the aim of promoting relaxation, reducing stress, and improving mental clarity.

6. Mindfulness: This technique involves paying attention to the present moment, with the aim of reducing stress and promoting relaxation.

In addition to these forms and techniques, Qigong also incorporates joint loosening exercises, stretching, and energy circulation exercises, helping to promote overall health and wellbeing.

By practicing Qigong forms and techniques regularly, we can improve our physical fitness and wellbeing, reduce stress and tension, and promote overall health and vitality. Whether you are interested in Tai Chi Qigong, Medical Qigong, or Daoist Qigong, there is a style of Qigong that can benefit you. With regular practice, Qigong can help promote overall health and wellbeing, leading to a happier, healthier life.

Five Animal Frolics

The Five Animal Frolics is a popular Qigong form that is based on the movements and behavior of five different animals - the tiger, deer, bear, monkey, and crane. This Qigong form is designed to promote physical fitness and wellbeing, while also improving mental clarity and reducing stress.

The Five Animal Frolics was first developed in China over 1,800 years ago by Hua Tuo, a famous physician and Qigong master. Hua Tuo observed the movements and behavior of different animals, and developed a series of exercises based on these observations, with the aim of promoting health and wellbeing.

Each animal in the Five Animal Frolics is associated with different physical and mental characteristics. The tiger, for example, is associated with strength and power, while the crane is associated with grace and flexibility.

Some common movements in the Five Animal Frolics include:

1. Tiger: This movement involves crouching down low to the ground, with the arms extended forward, and then springing up into a standing position. This movement is designed to promote strength and power, while also improving flexibility.

2. Deer: This movement involves standing on one leg, while lifting the other leg up and out to the side. This movement is designed to promote balance and coordination, while also improving circulation.

3. Bear: This movement involves crouching down low to the ground, with the arms extended forward, and then walking forward on the hands and feet. This movement is designed to promote strength and endurance, while also improving flexibility.

4. Monkey: This movement involves jumping up and down, while swinging the arms and legs. This movement is designed to promote agility and flexibility, while also improving circulation.

5. Crane: This movement involves standing on one leg, with the arms extended out to the sides, and then lifting the leg up and back behind the body. This movement is designed to promote balance and flexibility, while also improving circulation.

The Five Animal Frolics can be practiced by people of all ages and fitness levels. It is particularly popular among older adults, as it promotes physical fitness and mental clarity, while also reducing stress and promoting relaxation.

In addition to the physical movements, the Five Animal Frolics also incorporates breathing techniques and mindfulness exercises, helping to promote relaxation and focus, and preparing the mind and body for the demands of Qigong practice.

Eight Pieces of Brocade

The Eight Pieces of Brocade, also known as the Ba Duan Jin, is a popular Qigong form that has been practiced in China for over 1,000 years. This Qigong form is designed to promote physical fitness and wellbeing, while also improving mental clarity and reducing stress.

The Eight Pieces of Brocade consists of eight different movements, each designed to promote the flow of Qi, or life force energy, throughout the body. These movements are based on the traditional Chinese belief that the body contains twelve main meridians, or channels, through which Qi flows. The Eight Pieces of Brocade is designed to promote the flow of Qi through these channels, improving overall health and wellbeing.

Some common movements in the Eight Pieces of Brocade include:

1. Two Hands Hold up the Heavens: This movement involves standing with the feet shoulder-width apart, and raising the arms up overhead, with

the palms facing up. This movement is designed to promote the flow of Qi through the Lung meridian, promoting respiratory health.

2. Drawing the Bow to Shoot the Hawk: This movement involves standing with the feet shoulder-width apart, and pulling the arms back as if drawing a bow, while lifting one leg up off the ground. This movement is designed to promote the flow of Qi through the Gallbladder meridian, promoting liver health.

3. Separating Heaven and Earth: This movement involves standing with the feet shoulder-width apart, and reaching up with one hand while reaching down with the other hand. This movement is designed to promote the flow of Qi through the Spleen meridian, promoting digestive health.

The Eight Pieces of Brocade can be practiced by people of all ages and fitness levels. It is particularly popular among older adults, as it promotes physical fitness and mental clarity, while also reducing stress and promoting relaxation.

In addition to the physical movements, the Eight Pieces of Brocade also incorporates breathing techniques and mindfulness exercises, helping to promote relaxation and focus, and preparing the mind and body for the demands of Qigong practice.

The Eight Pieces of Brocade is considered one of the most fundamental Qigong forms, and is often used as a foundation for other Qigong practices. It is also used in traditional Chinese medicine as a way to promote health and wellbeing, and to treat a variety of physical and emotional ailments.

Six Healing Sounds

The Six Healing Sounds is a popular Qigong practice that has been used in China for centuries. This Qigong practice is designed to promote physical and emotional health by helping to release stagnant energy from the body and promote the flow of Qi, or life force energy.

The Six Healing Sounds involves making specific sounds while performing specific movements and postures, with the aim of stimulating and balancing different organs and meridians in the body. Each of the six sounds is associated with a different organ in the body, and is designed to promote the flow of Qi through that organ and its associated meridian.

Some common sounds and movements in the Six Healing Sounds include:

1. The sound "ssshhh" and the movement of placing the hands over the ears: This sound and movement is associated with the Kidneys, and is designed to promote the flow of Qi through the Kidney meridian.

2. The sound "haw" and the movement of rotating the neck: This sound and movement is associated with the Liver, and is designed to promote the flow of Qi through the Liver meridian.

3. The sound "hu" and the movement of raising the shoulders: This sound and movement is associated with the Lungs, and is designed to promote the flow of Qi through the Lung meridian.

The Six Healing Sounds can be practiced by people of all ages and fitness levels. It is particularly useful for those who experience stress, anxiety, and other emotional imbalances, as it helps to promote emotional stability and wellbeing.

In addition to the physical movements and sounds, the Six Healing Sounds also incorporates mindfulness and visualization techniques, helping to promote relaxation and focus, and preparing the mind and body for the demands of Qigong practice.

The Six Healing Sounds is considered one of the most effective Qigong practices for promoting overall health and wellbeing, and is often used in conjunction with other Qigong practices, such as Tai Chi and the Eight Pieces of Brocade.

Chapter Six

Qigong for Health and Healing

Qigong is a traditional Chinese practice that has been used for thousands of years to promote health and healing. This practice involves a combination of physical movements, breathing techniques, and mindfulness exercises, with the aim of promoting the flow of Qi, or life force energy, throughout the body.

Qigong can be used for a wide range of health and healing purposes, including:

1. Reducing stress and tension: Qigong is particularly effective at reducing stress and tension, as it promotes relaxation and mindfulness, and helps to release stagnant energy from the body.

2. Promoting physical fitness: Qigong can be used to promote physical fitness and improve flexibility, balance, and coordination.

3. Reducing chronic pain: Qigong has been shown to be effective at reducing chronic pain, particularly when used in conjunction with other medical treatments.

4. Improving emotional wellbeing: Qigong can help to promote emotional stability and wellbeing, reducing symptoms of anxiety, depression, and other emotional imbalances.

5. Boosting the immune system: Qigong has been shown to be effective at boosting the immune system, improving overall health and vitality.

There are many different forms of Qigong that can be used for health and healing purposes. Some popular forms of Qigong include:

6. Tai Chi: Tai Chi is a slow and gentle form of Qigong that is particularly effective at improving balance, flexibility, and coordination.

7. The Eight Pieces of Brocade: The Eight Pieces of Brocade is a popular Qigong form that is designed to promote physical fitness and wellbeing, while also improving mental clarity and reducing stress.

8. The Six Healing Sounds: The Six Healing Sounds is a Qigong practice that involves making specific sounds while performing specific movements and postures, with the aim of promoting the flow of Qi and promoting emotional wellbeing.

Qigong can be practiced by people of all ages and fitness levels. It is particularly useful for older adults, as it promotes physical fitness and mental clarity, while also reducing stress and promoting relaxation.

In addition to promoting overall health and healing, Qigong can also be used to treat specific medical conditions. Some conditions that can be treated with Qigong include:

9. High blood pressure: Qigong has been shown to be effective at reducing blood pressure in people with hypertension.

10. Chronic pain: Qigong can be used to reduce chronic pain, particularly when used in conjunction with other medical treatments.

11. Cancer: Qigong can be used to help manage the side effects of cancer treatment, such as fatigue and nausea.

Qigong for Stress Reduction

Stress is a common problem that affects millions of people around the world. It can cause physical and emotional symptoms, such as headaches, fatigue, anxiety, and depression. While there are many strategies for reducing stress, Qigong has been shown to be particularly effective at promoting relaxation and reducing stress levels.

Qigong is a traditional Chinese practice that involves a combination of physical movements, breathing techniques, and mindfulness exercises. It is designed to promote the flow of Qi, or life force energy, throughout the body, and is effective at reducing stress and tension.

Some common Qigong techniques for stress reduction include:

1. Deep breathing: Qigong involves deep breathing techniques, which help to slow down the heart rate, reduce blood pressure, and promote relaxation.

2. Mindfulness: Qigong involves mindfulness techniques, which help to focus the mind and reduce feelings of stress and anxiety.

3. Movement: Qigong involves gentle physical movements, which help to promote relaxation and reduce muscle tension.

Studies have shown that practicing Qigong regularly can lead to a significant reduction in stress levels. For example, a 2014 study published in the Journal of Alternative and Complementary Medicine found that practicing Qigong led to a significant reduction in stress and anxiety levels in participants.

Qigong can also be used in conjunction with other stress-reduction techniques, such as meditation and yoga. For example, a 2013 study published in the Journal of Psychiatric Research found that combining Qigong with mindfulness-based stress reduction led to a significant reduction in symptoms of depression and anxiety in participants.

One of the great things about Qigong is that it can be practiced by people of all ages and fitness levels. It is particularly useful for older adults, as it promotes physical fitness and mental clarity, while also reducing stress and promoting relaxation.

There are many different forms of Qigong that can be used for stress reduction. Some popular forms of Qigong for stress reduction include:

4. Tai Chi: Tai Chi is a slow and gentle form of Qigong that is particularly effective at promoting relaxation and reducing stress levels.

5. The Eight Pieces of Brocade: The Eight Pieces of Brocade is a popular Qigong form that is designed to promote physical fitness and wellbeing, while also improving mental clarity and reducing stress.

6. The Six Healing Sounds: The Six Healing Sounds is a Qigong practice that involves making specific sounds while performing specific movements and postures, with the aim of promoting the flow of Qi and promoting emotional wellbeing.

Qigong for Pain Management

Chronic pain is a common problem that affects millions of people around the world. While there are many strategies for managing pain, Qigong has been shown to be particularly effective at reducing pain levels and promoting healing.

Qigong is a traditional Chinese practice that involves a combination of physical movements, breathing techniques, and mindfulness exercises. It is designed to promote the flow of Qi, or life force energy, throughout the body, and is effective at reducing pain and improving physical function.

Some common Qigong techniques for pain management include:

1. Slow, gentle movements: Qigong involves slow, gentle movements that help to improve circulation, reduce muscle tension, and promote relaxation. These movements can be especially helpful for people with chronic pain, as they promote physical function and reduce pain levels.

2. Deep breathing: Qigong involves deep breathing techniques, which help to reduce stress levels and promote relaxation. This can be particularly helpful for people with chronic pain, as stress can exacerbate pain levels.

3. Mindfulness: Qigong involves mindfulness techniques, which help to focus the mind and reduce feelings of stress and anxiety. This can be particularly helpful for people with chronic pain, as stress and anxiety can exacerbate pain levels.

Studies have shown that practicing Qigong regularly can lead to a significant reduction in pain levels. For example, a 2015 study published in the Journal of Alternative and Complementary Medicine found that Qigong was effective at reducing pain levels in people with chronic low back pain.

Qigong can also be used in conjunction with other pain management strategies, such as physical therapy and medication. For example, a 2017 study published in the Journal of Pain Research found that combining Qigong with physical therapy led to a significant reduction in pain levels in people with knee osteoarthritis.

One of the great things about Qigong is that it can be practiced by people of all ages and fitness levels. It is particularly useful for older adults, as it promotes physical function and mental clarity, while also reducing pain levels.

There are many different forms of Qigong that can be used for pain management. Some popular forms of Qigong for pain management include:

4. Tai Chi: Tai Chi is a slow and gentle form of Qigong that is particularly effective at reducing pain levels and promoting healing.

5. The Eight Pieces of Brocade: The Eight Pieces of Brocade is a popular Qigong form that is designed to promote physical fitness and wellbeing, while also improving mental clarity and reducing pain levels.

6. The Six Healing Sounds: The Six Healing Sounds is a Qigong practice that involves making specific sounds while performing specific movements and postures, with the aim of promoting the flow of Qi and promoting emotional wellbeing.

Qigong for Immune System Support

The immune system is our body's natural defense against illness and disease. It plays a critical role in maintaining our overall health and wellbeing. While there are many strategies for supporting the immune system, Qigong has been shown to be particularly effective at boosting immune function and promoting overall health.

Qigong is a traditional Chinese practice that involves a combination of physical movements, breathing techniques, and mindfulness exercises. It is designed to promote the flow of Qi, or life force energy, throughout the body, and is effective at promoting immune system function.

Some common Qigong techniques for immune system support include:

1. Deep breathing: Qigong involves deep breathing techniques, which help to reduce stress levels and promote relaxation. This can be particularly helpful for immune system function, as stress can weaken the immune system.

2. Mindfulness: Qigong involves mindfulness techniques, which help to focus the mind and reduce feelings of stress and anxiety. This can be particularly helpful for immune system function, as stress and anxiety can weaken the immune system.

3. Movement: Qigong involves gentle physical movements, which help to improve circulation and promote overall health. This can be particularly helpful for immune system function, as improved circulation can help to distribute immune system cells throughout the body.

Studies have shown that practicing Qigong regularly can lead to a significant improvement in immune system function. For example, a 2015 study published in the Journal of Alternative and Complementary Medicine found that practicing Qigong led to a significant increase in immune system function in participants.

Qigong can also be used in conjunction with other immune system support strategies, such as healthy eating and good sleep hygiene. For example, a 2019 study published in the Journal of Traditional Chinese Medicine found that combining Qigong with dietary changes led to a significant improvement in immune system function in participants.

One of the great things about Qigong is that it can be practiced by people of all ages and fitness levels. It is particularly useful for older adults, as it promotes physical function and mental clarity, while also promoting immune system function.

There are many different forms of Qigong that can be used for immune system support. Some popular forms of Qigong for immune system support include:

4. Tai Chi: Tai Chi is a slow and gentle form of Qigong that is particularly effective at promoting immune system function and improving overall health.

5. The Eight Pieces of Brocade: The Eight Pieces of Brocade is a popular Qigong form that is designed to promote physical fitness and wellbeing, while also improving immune system function.

6. The Six Healing Sounds: The Six Healing Sounds is a Qigong practice that involves making specific sounds while performing specific movements and postures, with the aim of promoting the flow of Qi and promoting emotional wellbeing.

Chapter Seven

Advanced Qigong Practices

Qigong is a traditional Chinese practice that has been used for centuries to promote physical health, mental clarity, and spiritual development. While there are many forms of Qigong that are suitable for beginners and intermediate practitioners, there are also advanced Qigong practices that are designed for more experienced practitioners.

Advanced Qigong practices often involve a combination of physical movements, breathing techniques, and meditation exercises. They are designed to promote the flow of Qi, or life force energy, throughout the body, and to help practitioners achieve a deeper level of spiritual awareness and connection.

Some common advanced Qigong practices include:

1. Nei Gong: Nei Gong is an advanced form of Qigong that focuses on internal cultivation. It involves a series of physical movements and breathing techniques that are designed to open up the body's energy channels and promote the flow of Qi.

2. Dao Yin: Dao Yin is an advanced form of Qigong that focuses on alignment and balance. It involves a series of physical movements and postures that are designed to promote the flow of Qi and to help practitioners achieve a deeper level of physical and spiritual awareness.

3. Zhan Zhuang: Zhan Zhuang is an advanced form of Qigong that focuses on standing meditation. It involves holding specific postures for

extended periods of time, with the aim of promoting the flow of Qi and developing greater physical and spiritual strength.

Advanced Qigong practices are often taught by experienced Qigong masters, and require a high level of commitment and dedication from practitioners. They can take years of practice to master, and require a deep understanding of the principles of Qigong and the flow of Qi.

Despite their difficulty, advanced Qigong practices offer a wide range of benefits for practitioners. They can help to promote physical health, mental clarity, and spiritual awareness, and can provide a powerful tool for personal development and growth.

Some of the specific benefits of advanced Qigong practices include:

4. Improved physical strength and flexibility: Advanced Qigong practices can help to develop greater physical strength and flexibility, and can improve overall physical fitness.

5. Greater mental clarity and focus: Advanced Qigong practices can help to promote greater mental clarity and focus, and can help practitioners to achieve a deeper level of mindfulness and meditation.

6. Deeper spiritual connection: Advanced Qigong practices can help practitioners to achieve a deeper level of spiritual connection, and can promote a greater sense of inner peace and calm.

While advanced Qigong practices are not suitable for everyone, they can be a powerful tool for personal development and growth for those who are willing to dedicate the time and effort required to master them. With regular practice and the guidance of an experienced Qigong master, advanced Qigong practices can help practitioners to achieve greater physical health, mental clarity, and spiritual awareness.

Martial Qigong

Martial Qigong is a form of Qigong that is specifically designed for martial arts practitioners. It combines the physical movements and breathing techniques of traditional Qigong with the principles of martial arts, to help practitioners develop greater strength, flexibility, and focus.

Martial Qigong is based on the principles of Yin and Yang, and seeks to achieve balance and harmony in both the body and mind. It involves a series of physical movements that are designed to promote the flow of Qi, or life force energy, throughout the body, and to develop greater physical and mental strength.

Some common Martial Qigong techniques include:

1. Iron Shirt Qigong: Iron Shirt Qigong is a form of Martial Qigong that focuses on developing greater physical strength and resistance. It involves a series of physical movements and postures that are designed to strengthen the body's muscles and bones, and to promote overall physical fitness.

2. Tai Chi: Tai Chi is a form of Martial Qigong that is particularly effective at promoting balance and flexibility. It involves slow, fluid movements that are designed to promote the flow of Qi and to help practitioners achieve a deeper level of mental and physical relaxation.

3. Bagua Zhang: Bagua Zhang is a form of Martial Qigong that focuses on developing greater agility and flexibility. It involves a series of circular movements and footwork patterns that are designed to promote the flow of Qi and to help practitioners develop greater physical and mental focus.

Martial Qigong can be a powerful tool for martial arts practitioners of all levels. It can help to improve physical strength and flexibility, develop greater mental focus and concentration, and promote overall physical and mental health.

In addition to its physical benefits, Martial Qigong can also be an effective tool for self-defense. By promoting greater physical strength and mental focus, Martial Qigong can help practitioners to become more confident and effective in martial arts practice and in real-life situations.

Martial Qigong is often taught by experienced martial arts instructors, who are also trained in Qigong principles and techniques. These instructors can provide guidance and support to students, and can help them to develop a deeper understanding of the principles of Martial Qigong and its benefits for physical and mental health.

While Martial Qigong is primarily designed for martial arts practitioners, it can also be beneficial for anyone looking to improve their physical and mental health. By promoting greater physical strength and mental focus, Martial Qigong can help to reduce stress, improve overall fitness, and promote a greater sense of inner peace and calm.

Spiritual Qigong

Spiritual Qigong is a form of Qigong that is designed to promote spiritual development and growth. It involves a combination of physical movements, breathing techniques, and meditation exercises that are designed to promote the flow of Qi, or life force energy, throughout the body and to help practitioners achieve a deeper level of spiritual awareness and connection.

Spiritual Qigong is based on the principles of Taoism, which teaches that all living beings are interconnected and part of a larger whole. It emphasizes the importance of cultivating inner peace and harmony, and seeks to help practitioners achieve a deeper sense of spiritual connection and enlightenment.

Some common Spiritual Qigong techniques include:

1. Moving Meditation: Moving Meditation is a form of Spiritual Qigong that involves a series of physical movements and breathing techniques that are designed to promote the flow of Qi and to help practitioners achieve a deeper level of meditation and mindfulness.

2. Sitting Meditation: Sitting Meditation is a form of Spiritual Qigong that involves sitting in a meditative posture and focusing on the breath. It is designed to promote a deeper sense of inner peace and calm, and to help practitioners develop greater mental clarity and focus.

3. Visualization: Visualization is a form of Spiritual Qigong that involves visualizing positive images or thoughts. It is designed to help practitioners develop a deeper sense of spiritual connection and to promote greater mental and emotional balance.

Spiritual Qigong can be a powerful tool for personal growth and development. It can help practitioners to develop greater mental and emotional resilience, and to achieve a deeper sense of inner peace and calm. It can also be a powerful tool for overcoming negative thought patterns and habits, and for promoting greater overall health and wellbeing.

In addition to its spiritual benefits, Spiritual Qigong can also be effective in promoting physical health. By promoting the flow of Qi throughout the body, Spiritual Qigong can help to improve circulation, boost the immune system, and promote overall physical fitness.

Spiritual Qigong is often taught by experienced Qigong masters, who are trained in both the physical and spiritual aspects of the practice. These instructors can provide guidance and support to practitioners, and can help them to develop a deeper understanding of the principles of Spiritual Qigong and its benefits for personal growth and development.

While Spiritual Qigong is primarily designed for spiritual development and growth, it can also be beneficial for anyone looking to improve their physical and mental health. By promoting greater mental and emotional balance, Spiritual Qigong can help to reduce stress, anxiety, and depression, and to promote a greater sense of overall wellbeing.

Medical Qigong

Medical Qigong is a form of Qigong that is specifically designed to promote healing and wellness. It involves a combination of physical movements, breathing techniques, and meditation exercises that are tailored to the specific needs of individual patients, and are designed to promote the flow of Qi, or life force energy, throughout the body.

Medical Qigong is based on the principles of traditional Chinese medicine, and seeks to address the underlying causes of illness and disease by promoting the body's natural healing mechanisms. It can be used to treat a wide range of physical and emotional conditions, including chronic pain, digestive issues, respiratory problems, and anxiety and depression.

Medical Qigong practitioners use a variety of techniques to promote healing and wellness, including:

1. Qi emission: Qi emission is a technique in which the practitioner uses their own Qi to stimulate the flow of Qi in the patient's body. This can help to promote healing and balance in the body's energy systems, and can help to relieve pain and other symptoms.

2. Acupressure: Acupressure is a technique in which the practitioner uses pressure on specific points on the body to promote healing and balance.

It is based on the principles of traditional Chinese medicine, and is often used in conjunction with other Medical Qigong techniques.

3. Mind-body exercises: Mind-body exercises such as meditation and visualization can help to promote a deeper sense of relaxation and mental clarity, and can help to reduce stress and anxiety.

Medical Qigong can be a powerful tool for promoting health and wellness, and can be used to complement other medical treatments. It is often used in conjunction with acupuncture, massage therapy, and other forms of traditional Chinese medicine, and can be tailored to the specific needs of individual patients.

Medical Qigong practitioners are trained in both the physical and spiritual aspects of the practice, and are skilled in working with patients to identify the underlying causes of their conditions and to develop personalized treatment plans that address those causes.

Medical Qigong is often used to treat chronic conditions such as back pain, arthritis, and fibromyalgia, as well as conditions such as anxiety, depression, and insomnia. It can also be used to promote overall health and wellness, and to help prevent illness and disease.

In addition to its physical and emotional benefits, Medical Qigong can also be a powerful tool for spiritual growth and development. By promoting the flow of Qi throughout the body and balancing the body's energy systems, Medical Qigong can help practitioners to achieve a deeper sense of inner peace and connection.

Chapter Eight

Integrating Qigong into Daily Life

Integrating Qigong into daily life can have a powerful impact on overall health and wellbeing. Qigong is a form of Chinese exercise that involves a combination of physical movements, breathing techniques, and meditation exercises, and is designed to promote the flow of Qi, or life force energy, throughout the body. By incorporating Qigong into daily routines, individuals can experience a wide range of physical and mental benefits, including improved energy, reduced stress and anxiety, and greater mental clarity and focus.

Here are some tips for integrating Qigong into daily life:

1. Start with simple exercises: Qigong exercises can be simple and easy to learn, making them perfect for beginners. Start by learning a few basic exercises, such as the Five Animal Frolics or the Eight Pieces of Brocade, and practice them daily until they become part of your routine.

2. Practice in the morning: Many Qigong practitioners find that practicing in the morning is the most effective way to start the day. By practicing Qigong in the morning, individuals can set a positive tone for the day ahead and boost their energy levels.

3. Practice throughout the day: Qigong can be practiced at any time of day, and incorporating brief exercises throughout the day can help to maintain a sense of calm and balance. Take a few minutes to practice Qigong breathing exercises during a break at work or before bed.

4. Practice in nature: Qigong is often practiced outdoors, as the natural environment can help to promote a deeper sense of connection to the body and the natural world. Practice Qigong exercises in a park or natural setting, and focus on connecting with the energy of the earth and the sky.

5. Use Qigong to manage stress: Qigong can be a powerful tool for managing stress and anxiety. Incorporate Qigong breathing exercises into your daily routine, and use them as a way to calm the mind and promote relaxation.

6. Find a community: Practicing Qigong with others can be a powerful way to build community and support. Look for local Qigong classes or groups, and join a community of practitioners who share your interest in this ancient practice.

Integrating Qigong into daily life can have a powerful impact on overall health and wellbeing. By starting with simple exercises, practicing in the morning, throughout the day, and in nature, using Qigong to manage stress, and finding a community, individuals can experience the full benefits of this ancient practice.

Developing a Personal Qigong Routine

Developing a personal Qigong routine is an excellent way to reap the many benefits of this ancient Chinese practice. A personal Qigong routine can help to promote physical health, emotional balance, and spiritual wellbeing, and can be tailored to meet the specific needs and goals of individual practitioners.

Here are some tips for developing a personal Qigong routine:

1. Set goals: The first step in developing a personal Qigong routine is to set goals. What do you hope to achieve through your Qigong practice? Are

you looking to improve physical health, manage stress, or connect with your spiritual side? By setting clear goals, you can tailor your routine to meet your specific needs.

2. Choose exercises: There are many different types of Qigong exercises to choose from, including physical movements, breathing techniques, and meditation exercises. Choose exercises that align with your goals and preferences, and that you find enjoyable and engaging.

3. Start slowly: When starting a new Qigong routine, it's important to start slowly and build up gradually. Begin with just a few exercises, and gradually increase the duration and intensity of your practice as your body becomes more accustomed to the movements.

4. Incorporate mindfulness: Mindfulness is a key component of Qigong, and can help to promote a deeper sense of relaxation and mental clarity. Incorporate mindfulness techniques, such as deep breathing and visualization, into your routine, and focus on being present and fully engaged in your practice.

5. Practice regularly: Regular practice is essential for developing a personal Qigong routine. Aim to practice for at least 20-30 minutes per day, and try to practice at the same time each day to establish a routine.

6. Seek guidance: If you're new to Qigong or are unsure about how to develop a personal routine, seek guidance from a qualified Qigong practitioner. A qualified practitioner can provide guidance on exercises and techniques, and can help you to tailor your routine to meet your specific needs and goals.

By following these tips, individuals can develop a personal Qigong routine that promotes physical health, emotional balance, and spiritual wellbeing. Whether practicing for stress relief, improved energy, or spiritual growth, a personal Qigong routine can be a powerful tool for achieving greater health and happiness.

Qigong and Mindfulness

Qigong and mindfulness are two practices that are often used together to promote a deeper sense of relaxation, mental clarity, and spiritual growth. Qigong is a Chinese exercise system that combines physical movements, breathing techniques, and meditation exercises, and is designed to promote the flow of Qi, or life force energy, throughout the body. Mindfulness, on the other hand, is a practice that involves paying attention to the present moment, without judgment or distraction.

Here are some ways that Qigong and mindfulness can work together to promote greater health and happiness:

1. Increased awareness: Qigong and mindfulness both promote increased awareness of the body, mind, and spirit. By practicing Qigong exercises and mindfulness techniques, individuals can develop a greater sense of self-awareness, and can become more attuned to their thoughts, emotions, and physical sensations.

2. Deeper relaxation: Qigong exercises and mindfulness techniques can both be used to promote deep relaxation and a sense of calm. By focusing on the present moment and releasing tension from the body, individuals can experience a greater sense of peace and tranquility.

3. Improved mental clarity: Qigong and mindfulness can help to improve mental clarity and focus. By practicing Qigong exercises and mindfulness techniques, individuals can develop a greater sense of mental clarity and can become more productive and focused in their daily lives.

4. Spiritual growth: Both Qigong and mindfulness are often used as tools for spiritual growth and self-realization. By practicing Qigong exercises and mindfulness techniques, individuals can connect with their spiritual side and experience a greater sense of purpose and meaning in life.

5. Reduced stress: Both Qigong and mindfulness are effective tools for reducing stress and anxiety. By practicing Qigong exercises and mindfulness techniques, individuals can release tension from the body, calm the mind, and experience a greater sense of relaxation and wellbeing.

6. Improved physical health: Qigong exercises are designed to promote physical health and wellbeing, and can help to improve strength, flexibility, and balance. When used together with mindfulness techniques, Qigong can be a powerful tool for promoting overall physical health and wellbeing.

Qigong and Nutrition

Qigong is a Chinese exercise system that emphasizes the importance of balancing the body's energy, or Qi, through a combination of physical movements, breathing techniques, and meditation exercises. While Qigong is often associated with exercise, it is also closely linked to nutrition and the ways in which diet can impact the body's energy levels and overall health.

Here are some ways that Qigong and nutrition are interconnected:

1. Balancing Yin and Yang: In traditional Chinese medicine, foods are classified according to their energetic qualities, with some foods being considered "yin" (cooling and moistening) and others "yang" (warming and drying). Qigong emphasizes the importance of balancing yin and yang energies in the body, and a balanced diet can help to achieve this balance.

2. Eating for energy: Qigong emphasizes the importance of energy flow in the body, and a healthy diet can help to support this flow. Eating whole,

unprocessed foods that are rich in nutrients can help to nourish the body and provide sustained energy throughout the day.

3. Avoiding excess: In Qigong, excess is seen as a major cause of imbalance in the body. This includes excess consumption of food and drink, as well as excess emotions and thoughts. A balanced diet that avoids overeating and excess consumption of unhealthy foods can help to promote balance in the body.

4. Eating seasonally: In traditional Chinese medicine, it is believed that eating seasonal foods can help to support the body's natural rhythms and promote optimal health. Qigong practitioners may choose to eat seasonal foods in order to support their energy and overall health.

5. Eating mindfully: Qigong emphasizes the importance of mindfulness in all aspects of life, including eating. Mindful eating practices, such as savoring each bite and paying attention to hunger and fullness cues, can help to promote a healthy relationship with food and support balanced energy flow in the body.

In addition to these general principles, there are also specific foods and herbs that are commonly used in Qigong and traditional Chinese medicine to support overall health and wellbeing. For example, green tea is a popular beverage in Qigong, as it is believed to promote mental clarity and support energy flow in the body. Other foods and herbs that are commonly used in Qigong include ginseng, goji berries, and shiitake mushrooms, which are believed to have a range of health-promoting properties.

Chapter Nine

Qigong Resources and Further Study

Qigong is an ancient Chinese exercise system that focuses on the cultivation and balancing of Qi, or life energy, through a combination of physical movements, breathing exercises, and meditation techniques. For those who are interested in exploring Qigong further, there are a wealth of resources available that can provide guidance and support for deepening one's practice.

Here are some resources and avenues for further study for those interested in Qigong:

1. Qigong classes and workshops: The best way to learn Qigong is through a qualified instructor. Many communities have Qigong classes and workshops available, and these can be a great way to get started with the practice. In-person classes provide the opportunity to receive guidance and feedback from an experienced teacher, and can help to deepen one's understanding and connection to the practice.

2. Online courses and resources: For those who are unable to attend in-person classes, there are a variety of online courses and resources available for learning Qigong. These can range from pre-recorded videos to live virtual classes, and can be a great way to learn from the comfort of one's own home. Many Qigong instructors and organizations offer online resources, and there are also a number of online Qigong communities and forums where practitioners can connect and share knowledge.

3. Books and written resources: There are a multitude of books and written resources available on the topic of Qigong. These can range from introductory texts to more advanced and specialized resources. Some popular Qigong books include "The Way of Qigong" by Ken Cohen, "The Complete Idiot's Guide to T'ai Chi & Qigong" by Bill Douglas, and "The Root of Chinese Qigong" by Dr. Yang Jwing-Ming. These resources can be a great way to deepen one's understanding of Qigong theory and practice.

4. Qigong retreats and immersions: For those who are looking for a more immersive experience, there are a variety of Qigong retreats and immersions available. These can range from weekend workshops to longer-term retreats, and provide the opportunity to dive deeply into the practice and connect with like-minded individuals. Many retreats and immersions are held in natural settings, and may incorporate additional practices such as meditation, yoga, and mindfulness.

5. Qigong organizations and communities: There are a variety of Qigong organizations and communities around the world, which can provide support and resources for those interested in the practice. These organizations may offer events, resources, and networking opportunities, and can be a great way to connect with other practitioners and deepen one's understanding of Qigong.

6. Qigong DVDs and online videos: There are many Qigong DVDs and online videos available for those who prefer to learn through visual media. These can range from instructional videos to guided practices, and can be a convenient and accessible way to learn and deepen one's practice.

Finding a Qigong Teacher or Class

Qigong is an ancient Chinese practice that focuses on cultivating and balancing Qi, or life energy, through a combination of physical movements, breathing exercises, and meditation techniques. For those interested in deepening their Qigong practice, finding a qualified teacher or class can be an important step. Here are some tips for finding a Qigong teacher or class:

1. Research online: The internet can be a great resource for finding Qigong teachers and classes in your area. Many instructors and studios have websites or social media pages where they list their offerings, and there are also a variety of online directories and resources for locating Qigong classes. Some popular directories include Qigong Institute and MindBodyOnline.

2. Ask for referrals: If you know people who practice Qigong, ask them for recommendations for teachers or classes. Personal referrals can be a great way to find a teacher who is a good fit for you.

3. Check with local studios and wellness centers: Many yoga studios, martial arts schools, and wellness centers offer Qigong classes. Check with these types of establishments in your area to see if they offer Qigong classes, and to learn more about the instructors and their backgrounds.

4. Attend workshops and events: Qigong workshops and events can be a great way to learn more about the practice and connect with instructors and other practitioners. Attend local workshops or events to learn more about the practice and to meet potential teachers.

5. Look for a qualified instructor: When searching for a Qigong teacher or class, it's important to look for someone who is qualified and experienced. Look for an instructor who has completed a Qigong teacher training program and who has experience teaching students at your level. Check their credentials and ask for references if possible.

6. Consider the style of Qigong: There are many different styles and approaches to Qigong, and it's important to find a teacher or class that

aligns with your interests and goals. Some styles of Qigong may be more focused on health and wellness, while others may emphasize martial arts or spiritual development. Research different styles and approaches to find one that resonates with you.

7. Attend a class before committing: Before committing to a Qigong class or teacher, attend a class or two to get a feel for the teacher's style and approach. This can help you determine if the class is a good fit for you, and if the teacher is someone you feel comfortable learning from.

Recommended Books and Videos

For those interested in learning more about Qigong, there are a variety of books and videos available that can provide valuable information and guidance. Here are some recommended resources for those interested in deepening their Qigong practice:

Books:

1. "The Way of Qigong: The Art and Science of Chinese Energy Healing" by Kenneth S. Cohen - This classic book provides an in-depth introduction to the principles and practices of Qigong, including detailed instructions for a variety of exercises and techniques.

2. "Qigong Empowerment: A Guide to Medical, Taoist, Buddhist, and Wushu Energy Cultivation" by Liang Shou-Yu and Wu Wen-Ching - This comprehensive guide covers a wide range of Qigong practices, including healing, meditation, and martial arts.

3. "The Healing Promise of Qi: Creating Extraordinary Wellness Through Qigong and Tai Chi" by Roger Jahnke - This book offers practical guidance for incorporating Qigong and Tai Chi into daily life for improved health and wellbeing.

"The Complete Idiot's Guide to T'ai Chi & Qigong" by Bill Douglas - This beginner-friendly guide offers clear instructions and illustrations for a variety of Qigong exercises and techniques, along with helpful tips for practicing safely and effectively.

Videos:

"Qigong for Health and Vitality" with Lee Holden - This DVD offers a gentle, accessible introduction to Qigong for beginners, with a focus on promoting overall health and vitality.

"Qigong for Stress Relief" with Francesco Garripoli - This video provides guided instruction for a variety of Qigong exercises specifically designed to relieve stress and tension.

"Tai Chi & Qigong for Health" with Dr. Paul Lam - This DVD offers a comprehensive introduction to both Tai Chi and Qigong, with a focus on promoting physical health and mental wellbeing.

"Qigong for Beginners" with Mimi Kuo-Deemer - This gentle, beginner-friendly video provides clear instruction for a variety of Qigong exercises and techniques, with a focus on relaxation and stress relief.

In addition to these resources, there are also many online courses and classes available for those interested in learning Qigong. Many experienced teachers offer online classes and programs that can provide valuable guidance and support for those looking to deepen their practice.

Online Qigong Communities and Resources

In recent years, the internet has become a valuable resource for those interested in learning and practicing Qigong. Online Qigong communities and resources provide a convenient and accessible way for people all over the world to connect with others who share their interest in this ancient practice.

Here are some online Qigong communities and resources that can provide valuable support and guidance for those looking to deepen their Qigong practice:

The Qigong Institute - The Qigong Institute is a nonprofit organization dedicated to promoting Qigong research and education. Their website provides a wealth of information on the benefits of Qigong, as well as resources for finding Qigong classes and workshops.

Qigong Meditation and Healing - Qigong Meditation and Healing is a Facebook group dedicated to sharing information and resources related to Qigong. Members can connect with others who share their interest in Qigong and access a variety of articles, videos, and other resources.

Qigong for Healing - Qigong for Healing is an online community that provides support and resources for those using Qigong for healing purposes. Members can connect with others who are using Qigong to manage chronic illness, recover from injury, and promote overall health and well-being.

Qigong Association of America - The Qigong Association of America is a nonprofit organization that promotes the study and practice of Qigong in the United States. Their website provides information on Qigong research, classes, and certification programs.

Qigong Sensory Training Institute - The Qigong Sensory Training Institute is an online resource for those interested in developing their sensitivity to Qi. The website provides a variety of online courses and resources for learning to work with Qi energy.

In addition to these online communities and resources, there are also many Qigong teachers and practitioners who offer online classes and workshops. These can be a valuable way to deepen your practice and connect with others who share your interest in Qigong.

Chapter Ten

Specialized Qigong Practices

Qigong is a versatile practice that can be adapted to meet the needs and interests of different individuals. As a result, there are many specialized forms of Qigong that have been developed to address specific health issues, spiritual goals, and other areas of interest. Here are some examples of specialized Qigong practices:

Medical Qigong - Medical Qigong is a specialized form of Qigong that is focused on using the practice to promote healing and manage illness. Medical Qigong practitioners use Qigong exercises, meditation, and other techniques to work with Qi energy and support the body's natural healing processes.

Martial Qigong - Martial Qigong is a form of Qigong that is focused on developing physical strength, agility, and balance. This form of Qigong incorporates elements of martial arts training, and is often used by athletes and martial artists to enhance their performance.

Taoist Qigong - Taoist Qigong is a form of Qigong that is rooted in Taoist philosophy and spirituality. This form of Qigong is focused on developing a deep connection to the natural world and cultivating a sense of harmony and balance within the body and mind.

Buddhist Qigong - Buddhist Qigong is a form of Qigong that is rooted in Buddhist philosophy and spirituality. This form of Qigong is focused on developing mindfulness, compassion, and wisdom, and is often used as a tool for spiritual growth and self-transformation.

Women's Qigong - Women's Qigong is a specialized form of Qigong that is designed specifically for women's health and wellness. This form of Qigong incorporates exercises and meditation practices that are tailored to address issues such as menstrual cramps, hormonal imbalances, and menopause.

Children's Qigong - Children's Qigong is a form of Qigong that is adapted for the needs and interests of children. This form of Qigong incorporates playful exercises and activities to help children develop physical strength, emotional resilience, and mental focus.

Sports Qigong - Sports Qigong is a form of Qigong that is designed to enhance athletic performance. This form of Qigong incorporates exercises that are specifically targeted at improving agility, balance, coordination, and endurance.

Sound Qigong - Sound Qigong is a form of Qigong that incorporates the use of sound to work with Qi energy. This form of Qigong involves chanting or vocalizing specific sounds that are believed to have healing and transformative properties.

Zen Qigong - Zen Qigong is a form of Qigong that combines the practices of Zen meditation and Qigong. This form of Qigong is focused on cultivating a deep sense of presence, awareness, and connection to the natural world.

Specialized forms of Qigong can be a valuable way to tailor your practice to meet your specific needs and interests. By exploring different forms of Qigong and finding the one that resonates with you, you can deepen your practice and experience the many benefits of this powerful healing art.

Qigong for Women's Health

Qigong, an ancient Chinese practice that incorporates gentle movements, breathing techniques, and meditation, has been known to provide various health benefits. In particular, Qigong can be helpful for women's health concerns. Qigong is a holistic practice that aims to balance the body's energy, known as qi, and promote overall well-being. The practice can help improve physical, emotional, and mental health, and has been used to treat a range of health issues.

Women have unique health concerns that can be addressed with Qigong. In Traditional Chinese Medicine (TCM), women are believed to have a unique relationship with qi, as their bodies undergo cyclical changes every month. Qigong can help regulate these changes and promote balance in women's health. Here are some specific ways that Qigong can be beneficial for women's health:

1. Menstrual Health: Many women experience discomfort and pain during their menstrual cycle. Qigong exercises, such as abdominal breathing and gentle movements, can help alleviate these symptoms by promoting blood flow and energy circulation. Qigong can also help regulate the menstrual cycle by promoting balance and regulating hormonal imbalances.

2. Pregnancy and Postpartum Health: Qigong can help women during pregnancy by reducing stress and promoting relaxation. Qigong can also help prepare the body for labor and delivery by strengthening the pelvic floor muscles and promoting flexibility. After delivery, Qigong can help promote healing and recovery by reducing pain and stress.

3. Menopause: Menopause is a natural transition in a woman's life that can be accompanied by various symptoms, including hot flashes, night sweats, and mood changes. Qigong can help alleviate these symptoms by

promoting balance and reducing stress. Qigong exercises can also help strengthen the bones, which is particularly important for women who are at an increased risk of osteoporosis after menopause.

4. Breast Health: Qigong exercises, such as breast massage and gentle movements, can help promote breast health by improving blood and energy circulation. Qigong can also help alleviate breast tenderness and pain.

5. Emotional Health: Women are more likely than men to experience anxiety and depression. Qigong can help reduce stress and promote emotional well-being by calming the mind and balancing the body's energy.

When practicing Qigong for women's health, it is important to find a qualified instructor who has experience working with women's health concerns. It is also important to listen to your body and modify the practice as needed. Qigong can be practiced by women of all ages and fitness levels, making it an accessible and beneficial practice for women's health.

Qigong for Seniors

Qigong is an ancient Chinese practice that has been used for centuries to promote physical, mental, and spiritual health. It is a gentle and low-impact form of exercise that is especially well-suited for seniors. Below we will explore the benefits of qigong for seniors, as well as some of the specific qigong exercises that can be practiced to improve overall health and well-being.

One of the primary benefits of qigong for seniors is that it can help to improve balance and stability. As we age, our muscles and bones weaken, making falls and injuries more likely. Qigong exercises focus on improving the strength and flexibility of the body, which in turn can help to prevent falls and other accidents.

In addition to improving balance and stability, qigong can also help to reduce chronic pain and stiffness. Many seniors suffer from conditions such as arthritis and osteoporosis, which can make movement difficult and uncomfortable. By practicing qigong regularly, seniors can improve their flexibility and range of motion, which can help to reduce pain and stiffness.

Another benefit of qigong for seniors is that it can help to reduce stress and anxiety. Many seniors experience feelings of isolation and loneliness, which can contribute to anxiety and depression. Qigong exercises involve deep breathing and mindfulness, which can help to calm the mind and reduce feelings of stress and anxiety.

There are several qigong exercises that are particularly well-suited for seniors. One of the most popular is the Eight Brocades, which is a series of eight exercises that focus on improving overall strength and flexibility. Another popular exercise is the Five Animal Frolics, which is a series of movements based on the movements of five different animals.

In addition to these traditional qigong exercises, there are also specialized qigong practices that are designed specifically for seniors. For example, Chair Qigong is a modified form of qigong that can be practiced while sitting in a chair. This is an excellent option for seniors who have mobility issues or who are unable to stand for long periods of time.

It is important to note that while qigong is generally safe and low-impact, it is still important for seniors to consult with their healthcare provider before beginning any new exercise program. Seniors should also start slowly and gradually build up their qigong practice over time.

Qigong for Athletes and Sports Performance

Qigong is a Chinese practice that has been utilized for centuries to promote health, balance, and wellbeing. While often associated with traditional Chinese medicine and martial arts, it is also a valuable tool for athletes and sports performance. Below we will explore the benefits of Qigong for athletes and how it can be used to enhance athletic performance.

Qigong can be defined as a system of exercises and meditation designed to cultivate and balance the flow of Qi (vital energy) within the body. This practice has been shown to improve physical and mental health, reduce stress, and enhance overall wellbeing. Qigong is also a useful tool for athletes seeking to improve their performance on the field or court.

One of the primary benefits of Qigong for athletes is that it improves overall physical conditioning. Qigong exercises help to strengthen the body's core muscles, which are essential for athletic performance. These exercises can also increase flexibility, balance, and coordination, which are all important factors in athletic performance.

Another benefit of Qigong for athletes is that it can help to reduce the risk of injury. Qigong exercises are designed to improve the body's alignment and posture, which can help to prevent common injuries such as strains, sprains, and pulled muscles. Additionally, Qigong can help to improve circulation and reduce inflammation, which can further reduce the risk of injury.

In addition to physical benefits, Qigong can also help athletes to develop mental toughness and focus. Qigong meditation techniques help to quiet the mind and promote relaxation, which can be beneficial for athletes who need to maintain focus and concentration during competition. Furthermore, the discipline and focus required to practice Qigong can help athletes to develop mental toughness and resilience.

There are several Qigong techniques that are particularly useful for athletes. One technique is known as "Shaolin Qigong," which incorporates dynamic movements and deep breathing to strengthen the body and cultivate Qi. This technique is particularly useful for athletes who participate in high-intensity sports such as basketball, soccer, or football.

Another useful technique for athletes is "Tai Chi Qigong," which incorporates slow, flowing movements and deep breathing to improve balance, flexibility, and overall physical conditioning. This technique is particularly useful for athletes who participate in sports that require agility, such as gymnastics or martial arts.

One of the great advantages of Qigong is that it can be easily integrated into an athlete's existing training program. Qigong exercises can be performed in a variety of settings, including at home, in the gym, or even on the field or court. Additionally, Qigong exercises can be tailored to meet the specific needs of individual athletes, making it a versatile and customizable tool for improving athletic performance.

Chapter Eleven

Qigong and Emotional Health

Qigong is a practice that has been around for thousands of years and has been used to improve physical, mental, and emotional health. It is a type of mind-body exercise that combines movements, breathing techniques, and mental focus to help individuals achieve a state of relaxation and balance. Below we will explore the benefits of Qigong for emotional health.

Emotional health is an essential aspect of overall well-being, and Qigong can be an effective tool to promote emotional balance and reduce stress and anxiety. The practice of Qigong involves slow, gentle movements that can help calm the mind, reduce tension, and promote a sense of relaxation. This can be particularly helpful for individuals who struggle with negative emotions such as anxiety, anger, or sadness.

One of the key benefits of Qigong for emotional health is its ability to reduce stress levels. Stress is a common factor that can lead to emotional imbalances, and Qigong can be an effective way to manage stress levels. The deep breathing techniques used in Qigong help to oxygenate the blood, which can help to reduce cortisol levels, the hormone that is associated with stress. The gentle movements and mental focus used in Qigong can also help to release tension from the body and promote relaxation, which can further reduce stress levels.

Qigong can also be beneficial for individuals who struggle with anxiety. Anxiety can manifest in physical symptoms such as muscle tension, shortness of breath, and rapid heartbeat. Qigong can be an effective tool to help individuals manage these symptoms by promoting relaxation and reducing tension in the body. The slow, gentle movements of Qigong can help to promote a sense of calm, while the deep breathing techniques can help to regulate breathing and reduce feelings of panic.

In addition to reducing stress and anxiety, Qigong can also be helpful for individuals who struggle with depression. Depression can cause a range of emotional and physical symptoms, including fatigue, feelings of hopelessness, and loss of interest in activities. Qigong can be an effective way to help individuals manage these symptoms by promoting relaxation, reducing tension in the body, and promoting feelings of well-being. The practice of Qigong can also help individuals to develop a more positive outlook on life, which can be helpful in managing feelings of depression.

Another benefit of Qigong for emotional health is its ability to promote self-awareness and mindfulness. Qigong requires individuals to be fully present in the moment, focusing their attention on their breath and movements. This can help individuals to become more aware of their thoughts and feelings and develop a greater sense of self-awareness. The practice of Qigong can also help individuals to cultivate a more mindful approach to life, which can be helpful in managing stress and promoting emotional well-being.

Qigong can also be beneficial for individuals who have experienced trauma or other emotional challenges. The practice of Qigong can help individuals to release tension and negative emotions from the body, promoting a sense of calm and relaxation. The gentle movements of Qigong can also help to restore balance to the body's energy systems, which can be helpful in promoting overall emotional well-being.

Qigong for Anxiety and Depression

Qigong, an ancient Chinese practice that involves a combination of gentle movements, breathing techniques, and meditation, is gaining popularity as a complementary therapy for anxiety and depression. This mind-body practice has been shown to reduce stress, promote relaxation, and improve overall well-being, making it an effective tool for managing symptoms of anxiety and depression.

Qigong has its roots in traditional Chinese medicine and philosophy, which view the body and mind as interconnected systems. According to this philosophy, emotions and physical health are closely intertwined, and stress and negative emotions can lead to physical ailments. Qigong aims to balance the body's energy, or qi, by promoting the free flow of energy through the body's meridians or channels.

When practicing qigong, individuals focus on deep breathing, visualization, and gentle movements that help to release tension and promote relaxation. Qigong exercises can be practiced while standing, sitting, or lying down, making it accessible to individuals of all ages and fitness levels.

Several studies have shown that qigong can be effective in reducing symptoms of anxiety and depression. In one study, participants who practiced qigong for 12 weeks reported a significant reduction in symptoms of depression and anxiety compared to a control group that did not practice qigong. Another study found that qigong was effective in reducing symptoms of anxiety in patients with chronic obstructive pulmonary disease (COPD).

The benefits of qigong for anxiety and depression may be due to its effects on the body's stress response system. Qigong has been shown to reduce levels of the stress hormone cortisol and increase levels of the relaxation hormone oxytocin. This can lead to a reduction in feelings of anxiety and stress.

In addition to reducing stress, qigong can also improve mood and enhance overall well-being. Studies have shown that regular qigong practice can lead to improved quality of life, better sleep, and increased feelings of happiness and contentment.

It is important to note that while qigong can be an effective tool for managing symptoms of anxiety and depression, it should not be used as a substitute for professional medical treatment. Individuals with severe anxiety or depression should seek the guidance of a qualified healthcare professional.

Cultivating Emotional Balance Through Qigong

Qigong is a Chinese mind-body practice that emphasizes the cultivation of "qi" or life energy through breath, movement, and meditation. While it is often thought of as a physical exercise, qigong also has significant benefits for emotional health and wellbeing. Below we will explore how qigong can be used to cultivate emotional balance and resilience.

One of the primary ways that qigong supports emotional health is through its focus on breath and relaxation. In qigong practice, deep, slow breathing is used to help regulate the nervous system and promote a sense of calm and relaxation. This can be particularly beneficial for individuals who experience anxiety or high levels of stress. By learning to regulate the breath and relax the body, qigong practitioners can create a foundation of inner calm that supports emotional balance and stability.

In addition to regulating the breath, qigong also emphasizes the cultivation of "mindfulness," or present-moment awareness. Through mindful movement and meditation, qigong practitioners learn to focus their attention on the present moment, rather than getting lost in worries about the past or future. This can be particularly helpful for individuals who struggle with anxiety or depression, as it helps them to develop a greater sense of inner calm and groundedness.

Another important aspect of qigong for emotional health is its focus on cultivating positive emotions. Through specific movements and meditations, qigong practitioners learn to activate and enhance positive emotions such as joy, gratitude, and compassion. This can be particularly helpful for individuals who struggle with negative emotions such as anger, fear, or sadness. By learning to focus on positive emotions and cultivate a sense of inner joy and gratitude, qigong practitioners can create a more balanced and resilient emotional state.

Qigong also emphasizes the importance of developing a positive relationship with oneself and others. Through specific meditations and visualizations, qigong practitioners learn to cultivate self-compassion and compassion for others. This can be particularly helpful for individuals who struggle with feelings of self-doubt or low self-esteem, as it helps them to develop a more positive and supportive inner voice.

Finally, qigong can be a powerful tool for dealing with difficult emotions and experiences. Through specific meditations and movements, qigong practitioners learn to acknowledge and accept difficult emotions, rather than suppressing or avoiding them. This can be particularly helpful for individuals who have experienced trauma or other challenging life experiences. By learning to acknowledge and accept difficult emotions in a safe and supportive environment, qigong practitioners can develop greater emotional resilience and strength.

Qigong and the Five Elements

Qigong is a Chinese practice that involves physical movements, breathing techniques, and meditation to promote physical, mental, and spiritual health. One of the underlying concepts of Qigong is the five elements, which are an important aspect of traditional Chinese medicine and philosophy. The five elements, also known as Wu Xing, are Wood, Fire, Earth, Metal, and Water. Each element is associated with specific organs, emotions, and energy meridians in the body.

In Qigong, the five elements are used to create a harmonious balance in the body, mind, and spirit. The practice involves movements that activate and balance the energy associated with each element. By doing so, practitioners aim to achieve a state of internal balance that promotes overall health and well-being.

The Wood element is associated with the liver and gallbladder organs and is connected to the emotion of anger. The energy associated with Wood is said to be expansive and upward-moving. In Qigong, movements that activate the Wood element involve stretching and reaching upward, as well as movements that simulate chopping or cutting.

The Fire element is associated with the heart and small intestine organs and is connected to the emotion of joy. The energy associated with Fire is said to be expansive and outward-moving. In Qigong, movements that activate the Fire element involve circular arm movements and movements that simulate holding a ball of energy in the hands.

The Earth element is associated with the spleen and stomach organs and is connected to the emotion of worry. The energy associated with Earth is said to be stabilizing and centering. In Qigong, movements that activate the Earth element involve grounding and rooting movements, as well as movements that simulate gathering and holding energy in the center of the body.

The Metal element is associated with the lung and large intestine organs and is connected to the emotion of grief. The energy associated with

Metal is said to be contracting and inward-moving. In Qigong, movements that activate the Metal element involve movements that simulate drawing energy inward and upward, as well as movements that simulate pressing or squeezing.

The Water element is associated with the kidney and bladder organs and is connected to the emotion of fear. The energy associated with Water is said to be fluid and downward-moving. In Qigong, movements that activate the Water element involve movements that simulate flowing and spiraling, as well as movements that simulate diving or plunging.

In addition to the physical movements, Qigong also involves mental focus and visualization. Practitioners may visualize the energy associated with each element flowing through their body, or they may visualize a particular element as they perform the associated movements. This visualization helps to enhance the effectiveness of the practice and promote the desired internal balance.

Chapter Twelve

Qigong and Self-Cultivation

Qigong is a form of traditional Chinese exercise that involves physical movements, breathing techniques, and meditation. It has been practiced for thousands of years in China and is known to have numerous health benefits, such as reducing stress, improving flexibility, and boosting the immune system. However, qigong is not just a physical exercise, but also a practice that focuses on self-cultivation, personal growth, and spiritual development. Below we will explore how qigong can be used as a tool for self-cultivation.

In qigong, the term "self-cultivation" refers to the process of cultivating one's own physical, mental, and spiritual well-being through the practice of qigong. Self-cultivation is seen as an ongoing process of self-improvement and growth, and qigong is one tool that can be used to achieve this. The practice of qigong involves focusing on the breath, movement, and meditation, which can help to calm the mind, balance the emotions, and improve overall health.

One of the ways in which qigong can be used for self-cultivation is through the cultivation of "qi", or life energy. Qi is believed to flow through the body along energy channels called meridians, and qigong exercises are designed to help facilitate the flow of qi through these channels. By practicing qigong, one can learn to sense and control their qi, which can help to improve overall health and well-being.

Another way in which qigong can be used for self-cultivation is through the development of mindfulness. Mindfulness is the practice of being present and fully engaged in the present moment. When practicing qigong, one must be fully present in their body, breath, and movement, which can help to cultivate mindfulness. The practice of mindfulness can help to reduce stress, improve focus and concentration, and promote emotional well-being.

Qigong can also be used as a tool for self-cultivation by helping to develop self-awareness. Through the practice of qigong, one can become more aware of their body, breath, and thoughts. This increased self-awareness can help to identify areas of tension or imbalance in the body, which can then be addressed through qigong exercises. Additionally, increased self-awareness can help to improve emotional regulation, as one becomes more aware of their thoughts and emotions.

Finally, qigong can be used for self-cultivation by promoting a sense of inner peace and calm. The practice of qigong involves slow, gentle movements, and deep, rhythmic breathing, which can help to slow down the mind and promote relaxation. Through regular practice, one can cultivate a sense of inner peace and calm, which can help to improve overall well-being.

Qigong and Personal Development

Qigong, an ancient Chinese practice that involves movements, breath control, and meditation, has long been associated with physical and mental health benefits. However, the practice can also be used as a tool for personal development and growth.

At its core, Qigong is a mind-body practice that cultivates the flow of Qi, or life force energy, throughout the body. This can help to improve physical health, increase energy levels, and reduce stress and anxiety. However, the benefits of Qigong can extend beyond the physical realm, and the practice can be used to cultivate a deeper understanding of oneself and the world around us.

One way that Qigong can facilitate personal development is by helping individuals to develop greater self-awareness. By focusing on the breath, movements, and sensations of the body, Qigong practitioners are encouraged to become more attuned to their physical and mental states. This heightened awareness can help individuals to better understand their own thoughts and emotions, as well as how external factors such as stress or environment affect them.

Additionally, Qigong can help individuals to develop greater emotional intelligence. Through regular practice, individuals can learn to recognize and regulate their emotions, as well as become more empathetic and attuned to the emotions of others. This can lead to greater emotional stability, better relationships with others, and a more positive outlook on life.

Qigong can also be used to cultivate mindfulness and presence. Through the practice of meditation and breath control, individuals are encouraged to be fully present in the moment, and to let go of distractions or worries. This can help individuals to develop greater clarity of thought, reduce anxiety and stress, and cultivate a more positive attitude towards life.

In addition to these personal development benefits, Qigong can also help individuals to connect with a deeper sense of purpose and spirituality. The practice is deeply rooted in Chinese philosophy and spiritual traditions, and many Qigong practitioners incorporate these teachings into their practice. By exploring these philosophical and spiritual concepts, individuals can gain a greater understanding of themselves and their place in the world.

Furthermore, Qigong can help individuals to cultivate a greater sense of compassion and kindness towards others. By focusing on the flow of Qi and the interconnectedness of all things, practitioners are encouraged to cultivate a deeper sense of empathy and compassion for others. This can lead to greater altruism and a desire to contribute positively to the world.

Qigong and Creativity

Qigong, a traditional Chinese practice that combines physical movements, breathing techniques, and mental focus, has been linked to a variety of benefits, including increased physical and emotional health, improved concentration, and reduced stress. It's no wonder that Qigong has also been linked to creativity. Below we will explore the relationship between Qigong and creativity, and how practicing Qigong can help to foster creative thinking.

To understand the connection between Qigong and creativity, it's important to first understand the practice of Qigong itself. At its core, Qigong is about cultivating and balancing qi, or life energy, within the body. This is achieved through a combination of physical movements, deep breathing, and mental focus. The practice of Qigong is rooted in the belief that the body is made up of a network of energy channels, or meridians, and that the flow of qi through these channels is essential to maintaining physical and emotional health.

In Qigong, physical movements are carefully choreographed and coordinated with the breath, allowing the body to move in a fluid, flowing manner. This movement, combined with deep breathing, helps to increase oxygen flow and circulation, providing the body with more energy and vitality. Additionally, the mental focus required during Qigong practice can help to quiet the mind and reduce stress and anxiety.

It is believed that the increased energy and focus that result from Qigong practice can help to stimulate the creative mind. By increasing oxygen flow and circulation, Qigong can help to boost brain function and improve cognitive abilities. This can lead to improved concentration and focus, as well as increased creativity and problem-solving skills.

Furthermore, Qigong can help to balance the body's energy and reduce stress and anxiety, which can be major barriers to creativity. When we are stressed or anxious, our minds become preoccupied with worry and negative thoughts, making it difficult to think creatively or come up with new ideas. By reducing stress and anxiety, Qigong can help to clear the mind and make space for creative thinking.

There are also specific Qigong exercises that are designed to enhance creativity and mental clarity. For example, the Five Elements Qigong, which is based on the Chinese Five Elements theory, involves movements that are associated with each of the five elements (wood, fire, earth, metal, and water). By working with the elements and their corresponding energies, practitioners can stimulate creativity and improve mental clarity.

Another Qigong practice that can be helpful for creativity is the Lotus Meditation. This involves sitting in a cross-legged position and focusing on the breath while visualizing a lotus flower opening and closing. This meditation is believed to enhance creativity by increasing mental clarity and focus, and by promoting a sense of calm and tranquility.

In addition to these specific practices, simply incorporating regular Qigong practice into your routine can help to improve overall energy and vitality, which can have a positive impact on creative thinking. Regular practice can help to reduce stress and anxiety, improve concentration, and enhance mental clarity, all of which are essential for fostering creativity.

Qigong and Spiritual Growth

Qigong is an ancient Chinese practice that has been around for over 5000 years. It is an exercise system that combines physical movements, breathing techniques, and meditation to improve physical, emotional, and spiritual health. Qigong has many benefits, including improving energy levels, reducing stress, and boosting the immune system. One aspect of Qigong that has gained attention is its connection to spiritual growth.

1. The word "Qigong" is made up of two Chinese characters: "Qi" and "Gong." "Qi" refers to the life force energy that flows through all living things, while "Gong" means work or cultivation. Thus, Qigong is the practice of cultivating life force energy. This energy is also referred to as "prana" in Indian yoga and "ki" in Japanese martial arts.

Qigong helps people connect with the energy that flows within their bodies and the universe. The practice involves breathing exercises, movement, and meditation that stimulate the flow of Qi, allowing it to circulate more freely throughout the body. This improved circulation can lead to a feeling of greater vitality and a sense of connection to the world around us.

The spiritual aspect of Qigong is closely tied to its focus on mindfulness and meditation. In Qigong, practitioners are encouraged to cultivate a state of calm and awareness by focusing on their breath and movements. By doing so, they become more attuned to their inner world and their surroundings.

Through the practice of Qigong, individuals can develop greater self-awareness and a deeper understanding of their inner selves. This can lead to a greater sense of purpose and direction in life, as well as a greater sense of connection to the world around them.

In addition, Qigong can help individuals connect with their spirituality by providing a framework for exploring the deeper aspects of life. Many Qigong practitioners report feeling a greater sense of connection to the divine or a higher power through their practice.

Qigong can also help individuals develop qualities such as compassion, kindness, and forgiveness. Through its focus on mindfulness and meditation, Qigong can help individuals cultivate these qualities within themselves, leading to a greater sense of emotional well-being and a deeper connection to others.

Chapter Thirteen

Qigong for Chronic Conditions

Qigong is a traditional Chinese practice that has been used for thousands of years to promote health, healing, and well-being. It is based on the principle of balancing and cultivating the body's vital energy, or Qi. Qigong has been found to be particularly effective in managing chronic conditions, such as arthritis, asthma, and chronic pain.

The practice of Qigong involves a combination of gentle movements, breathing exercises, and mental focus. By practicing Qigong regularly, individuals can improve their overall physical and emotional health, reduce stress, and increase their sense of well-being.

Qigong has been found to be particularly effective in managing chronic pain. Chronic pain can have a significant impact on an individual's quality of life, making it difficult to perform daily tasks and engage in physical activity. Qigong has been shown to be effective in reducing pain and improving mobility in individuals with conditions such as arthritis and fibromyalgia. By practicing Qigong regularly, individuals can improve their strength, flexibility, and balance, which can help to reduce the risk of falls and other injuries.

Asthma is another chronic condition that can be effectively managed through the practice of Qigong. Asthma is a respiratory condition that causes the airways to become inflamed and narrow, making it difficult to breathe. Qigong has been found to be effective in improving lung function and reducing asthma symptoms in individuals with asthma. By practicing

Qigong regularly, individuals with asthma can improve their breathing, reduce the need for medication, and improve their overall quality of life.

In addition to managing chronic pain and asthma, Qigong has also been found to be effective in managing other chronic conditions, such as hypertension, diabetes, and heart disease. By improving the body's overall health and well-being, Qigong can help to reduce the risk of developing these conditions and improve the management of existing conditions.

Qigong is a safe and gentle practice that can be adapted to meet the needs of individuals of all ages and fitness levels. It is important to work with a qualified instructor who can provide guidance and support in developing a Qigong practice that is appropriate for your individual needs.

In addition to practicing Qigong, individuals with chronic conditions may also benefit from other lifestyle modifications, such as a healthy diet, regular exercise, and stress reduction techniques. By incorporating these strategies into their daily routine, individuals can improve their overall health and well-being, and better manage their chronic conditions.

Qigong for Arthritis

Qigong is a holistic practice that has been used for thousands of years in China for promoting health and healing. Qigong consists of a series of gentle movements, breathing techniques, and meditative practices that aim to balance the body's energy and improve overall health and well-being. One area where qigong has shown particular promise is in helping to manage chronic conditions such as arthritis.

Arthritis is a chronic inflammatory condition that affects the joints and causes pain, stiffness, and swelling. There are many different types of arthritis, including osteoarthritis, rheumatoid arthritis, and psoriatic arthritis, among others. While there is no known cure for arthritis, there are many different treatments available to help manage symptoms and improve quality of life. Qigong is one such treatment that has been shown to be effective in managing arthritis symptoms.

Qigong for arthritis typically involves a combination of movements, breathing techniques, and meditation. These practices are designed to increase circulation, reduce inflammation, and improve joint flexibility and range of motion. Qigong is a low-impact exercise that can be easily modified to suit different fitness levels, making it an ideal practice for those with arthritis who may have limited mobility.

One of the key benefits of qigong for arthritis is that it can help to reduce inflammation in the body. Inflammation is a major contributor to arthritis pain and stiffness, and reducing inflammation can help to alleviate these symptoms. Qigong has been shown to reduce levels of inflammation in the body by increasing circulation, improving lymphatic drainage, and promoting the release of endorphins, which are natural painkillers.

Another benefit of qigong for arthritis is that it can help to improve joint flexibility and range of motion. The gentle, flowing movements of qigong help to loosen up the joints and increase circulation to the affected areas. This can help to reduce pain and stiffness and improve overall mobility. In addition, the meditative aspects of qigong can help to promote relaxation and reduce stress, which can also contribute to improved joint function.

Qigong for arthritis can also be used as a complementary therapy alongside other treatments, such as medication and physical therapy. By combining different treatments, individuals with arthritis may be able to better manage their symptoms and improve their overall quality of life.

When practicing qigong for arthritis, it is important to work with a qualified instructor who can guide you through the movements and help you to modify the practice as needed to suit your individual needs. It is also important to listen to your body and not push yourself too hard, as this can exacerbate symptoms and lead to further injury.

Qigong for Diabetes

Qigong, a traditional Chinese practice, has been gaining popularity as a complementary therapy for diabetes management. It incorporates various techniques such as breathing, meditation, and gentle movements that can improve circulation, balance, and energy flow in the body. Diabetes, a chronic condition that affects millions of people worldwide, can cause several health complications if not managed properly. Below we will explore the benefits of Qigong for diabetes and how it can be an effective tool in diabetes management.

Firstly, Qigong helps in regulating blood sugar levels, which is a crucial aspect of diabetes management. Studies have shown that regular Qigong practice can lower fasting blood sugar levels, improve insulin sensitivity, and reduce the risk of diabetic complications. Qigong movements involve gentle stretching and contracting of muscles that stimulate the pancreas and promote insulin production. Furthermore, deep breathing techniques used in Qigong can lower stress levels, which can otherwise trigger a rise in blood sugar levels.

Secondly, Qigong can improve circulation and blood flow, which is essential for people with diabetes. Diabetes can cause poor circulation, which can lead to neuropathy, a condition that causes numbness and tingling in the feet and hands. Qigong exercises can help in improving circulation and reduce the risk of neuropathy. The gentle movements in Qigong, such as the Eight Pieces of Brocade, focus on stretching and strengthening the muscles in the legs, improving circulation in the lower extremities.

Thirdly, Qigong can help in managing diabetes-related complications. People with diabetes are at an increased risk of developing other health conditions such as cardiovascular disease, kidney disease, and retinopathy. Regular Qigong practice can improve cardiovascular health by reducing blood pressure, cholesterol levels, and improving blood flow. It can also help in improving kidney function and reducing the risk of retinopathy, a condition that can lead to blindness.

Fourthly, Qigong can help in weight management, which is crucial for people with diabetes. Obesity is a significant risk factor for type 2 diabetes, and weight management is an essential aspect of diabetes management. Qigong exercises, such as the Five Animal Frolics, focus on increasing flexibility, balance, and strength. It can also help in burning calories, improving metabolism, and promoting weight loss.

Lastly, Qigong can improve the overall quality of life for people with diabetes. Diabetes management can be a stressful and challenging task, and stress can further worsen diabetes. Qigong techniques such as meditation and deep breathing can lower stress levels, improve mood, and promote a sense of calmness and relaxation. Qigong can also improve sleep quality, which is essential for people with diabetes as lack of sleep can negatively impact blood sugar levels.

Qigong for Heart Health

Qigong is a mind-body practice that involves gentle movements, deep breathing, and meditation. It has been used for centuries in China as a means of promoting health, longevity, and spiritual growth. Recent studies have shown that qigong can be beneficial for heart health, reducing the risk of heart disease, lowering blood pressure, and improving overall cardiovascular function.

There are several qigong exercises and techniques that can be particularly helpful for improving heart health. One of the most commonly used is the "Five Animal Frolics" routine. This routine involves a series of movements that mimic the movements of different animals, including the tiger, deer, bear, monkey, and crane. Each movement is designed to stimulate different parts of the body, including the heart and cardiovascular system.

Another effective qigong exercise for heart health is "Standing Meditation". This involves standing in a relaxed, upright position and focusing on the breath. This practice helps to reduce stress and promote relaxation, which can be particularly helpful for reducing high blood pressure and other heart-related conditions.

"Tai Chi Qigong" is another practice that has been shown to be beneficial for heart health. This combines the gentle movements of tai chi with the deep breathing and meditation techniques of qigong. It has been shown to lower blood pressure, reduce cholesterol levels, and improve overall cardiovascular function.

"Ba Duan Jin" is another qigong exercise that can be helpful for heart health. This routine involves eight movements that are designed to stimulate different parts of the body, including the heart and lungs. It has been shown to improve cardiovascular function and reduce the risk of heart disease.

In addition to these exercises, there are several qigong techniques that can be particularly helpful for improving heart health. One of these is "Qi Gong for Heart Health and Blood Pressure", which involves deep breathing and visualization techniques to help reduce stress and improve cardiovascular function.

Another technique that can be helpful is "Qigong Breathing". This involves slow, deep breathing techniques that help to reduce stress and promote relaxation. It can be particularly helpful for reducing high blood pressure and other heart-related conditions.

Chapter Fourteen

Qigong and Energy Healing

Qigong is a traditional Chinese practice that is based on the principles of breathing, meditation, and movement. The aim of Qigong is to cultivate and balance the flow of Qi, or life energy, in the body. The practice is believed to promote physical, emotional, and spiritual well-being, and is often used in conjunction with other forms of traditional Chinese medicine, such as acupuncture and herbal remedies. One aspect of Qigong that is gaining popularity is its use in energy healing.

Energy healing is a form of complementary medicine that involves the manipulation of energy fields around the body to promote healing. Practitioners believe that blockages or imbalances in these energy fields can lead to illness or disease. Energy healing techniques aim to remove these blockages and restore balance to the body's energy fields, thus promoting healing.

Qigong is often used as an energy healing technique because it is believed to be effective in balancing the flow of Qi in the body. In Qigong, practitioners use specific movements, breathing techniques, and meditation to cultivate and circulate Qi throughout the body. By doing so, it is believed that the body's energy fields can be balanced and blockages can be removed, allowing for the free flow of Qi and promoting health and well-being.

One Qigong technique that is often used in energy healing is known as Qi emission or external Qi healing. This technique involves the use of a Qigong practitioner to emit Qi to a patient in order to balance their energy fields and promote healing. The practitioner uses specific movements and breathing techniques to cultivate and circulate Qi in their own body, before directing it towards the patient. The patient may feel sensations of warmth or tingling as the Qi is directed towards them.

Another Qigong technique that is used in energy healing is known as self-cultivation. This technique involves the use of Qigong to cultivate one's own Qi, in order to promote self-healing. Practitioners use specific movements, breathing techniques, and meditation to cultivate and circulate Qi throughout their own body. By doing so, it is believed that blockages can be removed and balance can be restored to the body's energy fields, promoting health and well-being.

In addition to these techniques, Qigong is also believed to be effective in treating specific conditions through energy healing. For example, Qigong has been used to treat chronic pain, including back pain and arthritis. It is believed that by restoring balance to the body's energy fields, pain and inflammation can be reduced. Qigong has also been used to treat depression, anxiety, and other emotional disorders. By promoting relaxation and reducing stress, Qigong is believed to improve mood and promote emotional well-being.

Qigong and Reiki

Qigong and Reiki are two practices that are often used together in holistic healing, energy work, and spiritual growth. Both practices are rooted in ancient Eastern traditions and have gained popularity in the West over the past few decades. While they have some similarities, they also have distinct differences that make each practice unique.

Qigong, also known as chi kung, is a Chinese practice that involves the cultivation and balance of energy, or chi, through gentle movements, breathing techniques, and meditation. It is based on the principles of Traditional Chinese Medicine (TCM) and the concept of qi, which is the life force or vital energy that flows through all living things. Qigong is often used as a form of exercise, meditation, and self-healing, and is believed to promote physical, mental, and spiritual well-being.

Reiki, on the other hand, is a Japanese practice that involves the use of healing energy channeled through the hands. It was developed by Mikao Usui in the early 20th century and is based on the belief that the practitioner can tap into the universal life force energy and use it to promote healing and balance in the body, mind, and spirit. Reiki is often used to alleviate physical and emotional pain, reduce stress and anxiety, and promote relaxation and overall well-being.

While both practices focus on the cultivation and balancing of energy, they differ in their approach and techniques. Qigong involves physical movements, such as slow and fluid stretches and postures, along with breathing techniques and meditation. It is a more active practice that can be used for both exercise and meditation. Reiki, on the other hand, is a more passive practice that involves the practitioner placing their hands on or near the body to channel healing energy. It is often used as a complement to other healing practices, such as massage or acupuncture.

In terms of their benefits, both Qigong and Reiki are believed to promote physical, mental, and spiritual well-being. Qigong has been shown to improve balance, flexibility, and strength, reduce stress and anxiety, and alleviate symptoms of chronic conditions such as arthritis and diabetes. It is also believed to promote mental clarity and spiritual growth. Reiki is believed to promote relaxation, reduce pain and inflammation, and alleviate symptoms of anxiety and depression. It is also used to promote spiritual growth and a deeper connection to the self and the universe.

For those interested in learning Qigong or Reiki, there are many resources available. Qigong classes can often be found at community centers, yoga studios, and martial arts schools. There are also many online resources, such as videos and tutorials, that can be used to learn Qigong from home. Reiki practitioners can be found through directories or by word of mouth. Many practitioners offer private sessions, and there are also classes available for those interested in becoming a certified Reiki practitioner.

Qigong and Chakra Balancing

Qigong is an ancient Chinese practice that has been used for centuries to cultivate and balance one's energy, or Qi. Chakra balancing is another energy-based practice that originated in India and is based on the idea that there are seven energy centers, or chakras, in the body that need to be in balance in order to promote overall well-being. Both practices share the goal of promoting balance and harmony within the body and mind, making them a natural complement to each other.

In Qigong, the focus is on cultivating and moving one's Qi through various exercises, postures, and meditations. This is achieved through various techniques such as deep breathing, visualization, and physical movements designed to stimulate and circulate the Qi throughout the body. By doing so, the body's natural healing abilities are enhanced, and the body and mind are brought into a state of balance and harmony.

Chakra balancing, on the other hand, is based on the idea that the body has seven chakras that are responsible for different aspects of one's physical, emotional, and spiritual well-being. Each chakra is associated with a specific color, sound, and element, and when these chakras are out of balance, it can lead to physical or emotional imbalances. Chakra balancing techniques aim to bring these energy centers back into balance through a variety of methods such as meditation, visualization, and energy work.

There are several ways in which Qigong and chakra balancing can work together to enhance one's overall well-being. For example, Qigong exercises can help to stimulate and balance the flow of energy in the body, which can help to bring the chakras into balance. Similarly, chakra balancing techniques can help to address imbalances in specific chakras that may be contributing to physical or emotional issues, which can be further supported by the practice of Qigong.

Some Qigong exercises and practices can also be specifically targeted towards balancing certain chakras. For example, the practice of "Inner Smile Meditation" in Qigong is often used to bring balance to the heart chakra, which is associated with love, compassion, and forgiveness. Similarly, certain physical movements in Qigong, such as those that involve twisting or rotating the spine, can help to stimulate the energy flow in the solar plexus chakra, which is associated with personal power and self-esteem.

Qigong and Distance Healing

Qigong is an ancient Chinese practice that involves the coordination of movement, breath, and meditation for the purposes of enhancing physical and mental health. One of the lesser-known applications of qigong is distance healing, which involves sending energy or qi to someone who is not physically present. Below we will explore the principles behind qigong distance healing and its potential benefits.

Qigong distance healing is based on the principles of traditional Chinese medicine, which views health as a balance of energy or qi in the body. According to this theory, physical or emotional ailments arise when the flow of qi is disrupted or blocked. By practicing qigong, individuals can cultivate and balance their own qi, which can then be used to help others.

In distance healing, the practitioner uses visualization techniques to send qi to the recipient. The practitioner first enters a meditative state and imagines a connection between themselves and the recipient. They then visualize sending healing energy to the recipient, focusing on specific areas of the body or emotional states that may be causing discomfort.

While there is limited scientific research on the efficacy of distance healing, anecdotal evidence suggests that it can be beneficial for a variety of conditions. For example, some individuals report feeling a sense of relaxation and peace after a distance healing session, while others report improvements in physical symptoms such as pain or inflammation. It is important to note, however, that distance healing should not be used as a replacement for conventional medical treatment.

One potential benefit of qigong distance healing is that it can be practiced from anywhere, making it accessible to individuals who may not have access to in-person healing practices. Additionally, distance healing can be useful for individuals who are unable to physically attend a healing session due to illness or injury.

In order to practice qigong distance healing effectively, it is important to have a strong foundation in qigong practice. This involves developing a regular qigong routine and cultivating awareness of one's own energy and the energy of others. It is also important to approach distance healing with a sense of compassion and an intention to help others, rather than seeking personal gain.

In addition to distance healing, qigong can also be used in combination with other energy healing practices such as reiki or chakra balancing. These practices share similar principles and can be complementary in supporting overall health and well-being.

Chapter Fifteen

Qigong for Better Sleep

Qigong, an ancient Chinese practice of cultivating life energy or qi, has been known to offer a wide range of health benefits, including improved sleep quality. For individuals suffering from insomnia or other sleep disorders, practicing Qigong can be a simple yet effective way to promote better sleep.

Qigong involves gentle movements, breathing techniques, and meditation, all of which help to relax the mind and body. By practicing Qigong regularly, one can reduce stress, alleviate tension, and improve overall well-being, which can all contribute to a better night's sleep.

One of the key benefits of Qigong is its ability to calm the mind and reduce stress. Stress is a common cause of insomnia and other sleep disorders, and it can prevent the body from entering a deep and restful state of sleep. By practicing Qigong, individuals can learn to regulate their breathing, reduce tension in the body, and clear their minds of distracting thoughts. This can help to reduce stress and anxiety, making it easier to fall asleep and stay asleep.

Another way in which Qigong can improve sleep quality is by regulating the body's circadian rhythm. The circadian rhythm is the body's internal clock that regulates sleep and wake cycles. When the circadian rhythm is disrupted, it can lead to sleep disorders and other health problems. Qigong helps to balance the body's energy, which can in turn regulate the circadian rhythm and promote a more natural sleep cycle.

Additionally, Qigong can help to alleviate physical discomfort that may interfere with sleep. Chronic pain, discomfort, and tension in the body can make it difficult to fall asleep and stay asleep. By practicing Qigong, individuals can stretch and loosen their muscles, improve circulation, and release tension in the body. This can help to alleviate physical discomfort and promote a more relaxed state, making it easier to fall asleep and stay asleep throughout the night.

There are many different Qigong exercises that can be beneficial for improving sleep quality. Some of the most popular techniques include abdominal breathing, which involves breathing deeply and slowly from the diaphragm; the Five Animal Frolics, which involves movements inspired by the movements of animals; and the Eight Pieces of Brocade, which is a series of exercises designed to strengthen and loosen the body. These exercises can be practiced alone or as part of a structured Qigong routine.

In addition to practicing Qigong exercises, individuals can also incorporate Qigong principles into their daily life to promote better sleep. For example, one can practice deep breathing and relaxation techniques before bedtime, avoid consuming caffeine or alcohol in the evening, and establish a regular sleep schedule. By integrating these principles into their daily routine, individuals can create a healthy sleep environment and promote better sleep quality.

It is important to note that Qigong is not a substitute for medical treatment for sleep disorders. Individuals who are experiencing chronic insomnia or other sleep disorders should seek the advice of a healthcare professional. However, Qigong can be a useful complementary therapy for improving sleep quality and promoting overall well-being.

Qigong Techniques for Relaxation and Calm

Qigong is an ancient Chinese practice that involves a series of physical movements, meditation, and breathing techniques to promote physical, mental, and emotional well-being. One of the main benefits of qigong is its ability to induce relaxation and calm, making it an ideal practice for reducing stress and anxiety.

Qigong has been used for centuries to improve overall health and well-being, and its benefits have been scientifically proven. Studies have shown that practicing qigong can help reduce stress, anxiety, and depression, and improve mood and sleep quality.

There are several qigong techniques that are specifically designed to promote relaxation and calm. One of the most common techniques is known as the "Four-Part Breath". This technique involves taking a deep breath in through the nose, holding it for a few seconds, exhaling slowly through the mouth, and then holding the breath out for a few seconds before taking another deep breath in. This technique can be repeated several times, and is often used at the beginning of a qigong practice to help calm the mind and body.

Another qigong technique that is effective for inducing relaxation is known as "Shaking Qigong". This technique involves standing with your feet shoulder-width apart, and shaking your body from head to toe. The shaking motion helps to release tension and stress from the body, and can be done for several minutes at a time.

"Meditative Qigong" is another technique that is effective for promoting relaxation and calm. This technique involves standing or sitting in a relaxed position and focusing on your breath. You can also visualize a peaceful scene or repeat a positive affirmation to help calm your mind and promote relaxation.

"Tai Chi Qigong" is a form of qigong that involves slow, flowing movements that promote relaxation and calm. This technique is often used in combination with meditation and deep breathing to help reduce stress and anxiety.

In addition to these techniques, there are also specific qigong exercises that are designed to promote relaxation and calm. One of these exercises is known as "Kidney Breathing". This exercise involves standing with your feet shoulder-width apart, placing your hands on your lower back, and taking deep breaths while focusing on the sensation of your breath in your kidneys.

Another exercise that is effective for promoting relaxation is known as "Sitting Qigong". This exercise involves sitting in a relaxed position and focusing on your breath. You can also visualize a peaceful scene or repeat a positive affirmation to help calm your mind and promote relaxation.

Qigong and Insomnia

Qigong is an ancient Chinese practice that combines physical movement, meditation, and breathing exercises to improve physical and mental health. Qigong has been found to be effective in treating many health conditions, including insomnia.

Insomnia is a sleep disorder characterized by difficulty falling or staying asleep. It can lead to daytime fatigue, irritability, and decreased productivity. There are many factors that can contribute to insomnia, such as stress, anxiety, depression, and physical pain. Insomnia can also be a side effect of medications or other medical conditions.

Qigong can be an effective way to treat insomnia because it helps to reduce stress and anxiety, which are often the main causes of sleep difficulties.

Qigong can also help to improve the flow of Qi, or vital energy, throughout the body. When Qi is flowing smoothly, the body is better able to relax and sleep.

There are several Qigong techniques that can be used to help alleviate insomnia. One of the most effective techniques is called the "Four-Part Deep Breathing" exercise. This exercise involves inhaling deeply through the nose, filling the lungs with air, and holding the breath for a few seconds before exhaling slowly through the mouth. This exercise can help to calm the mind and relax the body, making it easier to fall asleep.

Another effective Qigong technique for insomnia is the "Inner Smile" meditation. This meditation involves focusing on positive emotions and feelings, such as love, joy, and happiness, and directing them inward toward the body. This can help to reduce stress and anxiety, which can be major factors in sleep difficulties.

The "Eight Pieces of Brocade" is another Qigong practice that can be helpful for insomnia. This practice involves a series of gentle movements and stretches that help to improve circulation and reduce tension in the body. This can help to alleviate physical pain and discomfort, which can often make it difficult to sleep.

It is important to note that Qigong should not be used as a substitute for medical treatment for insomnia. If you are experiencing chronic insomnia, it is important to speak with a healthcare professional to determine the underlying cause and develop a treatment plan.

In addition to Qigong techniques, there are several other lifestyle changes that can be helpful for improving sleep. These include establishing a regular sleep schedule, avoiding caffeine and alcohol before bedtime, and creating a comfortable sleep environment.

Qigong and Sleep Quality

Qigong is an ancient Chinese practice that involves movement, meditation, and breath control to cultivate energy, improve health, and promote spiritual growth. In recent years, qigong has gained popularity as a natural and holistic approach to treating sleep disorders and improving sleep quality. Below we will explore the ways in which qigong can be used to improve sleep quality and the scientific evidence supporting its effectiveness.

Sleep is essential for maintaining good health, and chronic sleep deprivation can lead to a range of physical and mental health problems. Insomnia is a common sleep disorder characterized by difficulty falling asleep, staying asleep, or waking up too early. It affects up to 30% of the population and can have a significant impact on daily life, including mood, energy levels, and productivity. Qigong is a safe and effective way to address the underlying causes of insomnia and promote better sleep quality.

One of the ways qigong improves sleep quality is by reducing stress and promoting relaxation. Stress is a common cause of sleep disturbances and can interfere with the body's natural sleep-wake cycle. Qigong involves slow, gentle movements, deep breathing, and mindfulness meditation, which help to calm the mind and relax the body. This can help to reduce stress levels and promote a sense of inner peace and tranquility, which is essential for good sleep.

Another way qigong can improve sleep quality is by increasing the flow of Qi or energy throughout the body. In Chinese medicine, insomnia is often attributed to an imbalance of Qi or an obstruction in the flow of energy. Qigong involves gentle movements that stretch and strengthen the muscles, increase circulation, and stimulate the flow of energy through the body's meridians. By promoting the free flow of Qi, qigong can help to improve sleep quality and relieve insomnia.

Qigong can also improve sleep quality by promoting physical relaxation. When we are tense, our muscles can become stiff and sore, which can make it difficult to get comfortable and fall asleep. Qigong involves gentle stretching and movement that can help to release tension and relax the muscles. This can promote physical relaxation, making it easier to fall asleep and stay asleep.

There is scientific evidence to support the use of qigong for improving sleep quality. A study published in the Journal of Alternative and Complementary Medicine found that practicing qigong for 12 weeks led to significant improvements in sleep quality, including increased total sleep time, improved sleep efficiency, and reduced sleep disturbances. Another study published in the Journal of Sleep Research found that practicing qigong for six months led to significant improvements in subjective sleep quality, sleep latency, and sleep duration.

Qigong can be practiced in many different ways to promote better sleep quality. One simple and effective technique is called the "Sleeping Qigong" or "Sleeping Tiger Qigong." This technique involves lying down in a comfortable position and focusing on slow, deep breathing while visualizing the body's energy flowing freely and smoothly. This technique is especially effective for promoting physical relaxation and reducing stress levels, making it an ideal practice for people with insomnia.

Chapter Sixteen

Qigong and Workplace Wellness

Qigong, an ancient Chinese practice, has been gaining popularity in recent years as a method of promoting health and wellness. One area where it has shown promise is in workplace wellness programs. Below we will explore how Qigong can be incorporated into workplace wellness initiatives to improve employee health, productivity, and job satisfaction.

Qigong is a holistic practice that involves gentle movements, breathing techniques, and meditation. It is based on the belief that the body is a system of energy channels, or meridians, and that by practicing Qigong, one can stimulate and balance the flow of energy, or Qi, throughout the body. This can lead to improved physical health, reduced stress, and increased mental clarity.

One of the main benefits of Qigong is its ability to reduce stress. Stress is a common problem in the workplace, and it can have serious negative effects on employee health and productivity. Qigong's emphasis on breathing and relaxation techniques can help employees manage stress more effectively, leading to a calmer, more focused work environment.

Qigong can also improve physical health, which is another important aspect of workplace wellness. The gentle movements of Qigong can help improve flexibility, balance, and coordination, as well as reduce pain and stiffness in the muscles and joints. This can be particularly beneficial for employees who work in jobs that require repetitive motions or sitting for long periods of time.

In addition to physical and mental benefits, Qigong can also promote spiritual wellness. Many Qigong practices include meditation and visualization techniques that can help employees connect with their inner selves and find a greater sense of purpose and meaning in their work.

So how can Qigong be incorporated into workplace wellness programs? One approach is to offer Qigong classes or workshops for employees. These can be taught by certified Qigong instructors or by employees who have been trained in Qigong techniques. Classes can be offered before or after work or during lunch breaks, and can be tailored to different levels of experience and physical ability.

Another approach is to incorporate Qigong into existing wellness initiatives. For example, employers can encourage employees to take short Qigong breaks throughout the day, where they can practice simple Qigong movements and breathing techniques to help reduce stress and improve focus. Qigong can also be incorporated into mindfulness or meditation programs, where employees can learn to use Qigong techniques to enhance their practice.

Employers can also provide resources and materials on Qigong for employees to access on their own time. This could include instructional videos, books, or online courses that employees can use to learn about Qigong and develop their own practice.

It's worth noting that incorporating Qigong into workplace wellness programs requires a certain level of commitment from both employers and employees. Employers need to be willing to invest in Qigong classes or workshops, and employees need to be motivated to participate and make Qigong a regular part of their routine. However, the potential benefits to both individual employees and the workplace as a whole make it a worthwhile investment.

Qigong Exercises for Office Workers

Qigong is a Chinese practice that involves physical movements, breathing techniques, and meditation. It is a form of exercise that has been practiced for thousands of years and has numerous health benefits. One of the benefits of Qigong is that it can be practiced by people of all ages and fitness levels, including office workers who spend most of their time sitting at a desk. Below we will explore Qigong exercises that office workers can practice to improve their health and well-being.

One of the main problems that office workers face is a sedentary lifestyle, which can lead to various health problems such as obesity, heart disease, and diabetes. Qigong can help counteract the negative effects of a sedentary lifestyle by promoting movement and circulation. Here are some Qigong exercises that office workers can practice at their desk:

Seated Spinal Twist

The Seated Spinal Twist is a simple exercise that can help relieve tension in the back and neck. To perform this exercise, sit up straight in your chair with your feet flat on the ground. Place your left hand on your right knee and twist your torso to the right. Hold the stretch for a few breaths and then repeat on the other side.

Shoulder Rolls

Shoulder Rolls are a great way to relieve tension in the shoulders and neck. To perform this exercise, sit up straight in your chair and roll your shoulders forward and backward in a circular motion. Repeat for a few minutes, then switch directions.

Chest Opener

The Chest Opener is an excellent exercise for people who spend a lot of time sitting in front of a computer. It helps to stretch the chest muscles and improve posture. To perform this exercise, sit up straight in your chair and interlace your fingers behind your back. Gently lift your hands away from your back and hold the stretch for a few breaths.

Desk Push-Ups

Desk Push-Ups are a great way to strengthen the chest, arms, and core muscles. To perform this exercise, stand up in front of your desk and place your hands on the edge of the desk, shoulder-width apart. Step your feet back until your body is in a straight line, then bend your elbows and lower your chest toward the desk. Push back up to the starting position and repeat for 10-15 repetitions.

Leg Raises

Leg Raises are a simple exercise that can help improve circulation in the legs and lower back. To perform this exercise, sit up straight in your chair and raise one leg off the ground, keeping it straight. Hold the leg up for a few breaths and then lower it back down. Repeat on the other side.

Standing Stretch

The Standing Stretch is a great way to stretch the entire body and increase circulation. To perform this exercise, stand up and raise your arms above your head, interlacing your fingers. Gently lean to one side, stretching the opposite side of your body. Hold the stretch for a few breaths and then repeat on the other side.

Mindful Breathing

Mindful Breathing is a technique that can help reduce stress and increase focus. To practice this technique, sit up straight in your chair and close your eyes. Take a few deep breaths, inhaling through your nose and exhaling through your mouth. Focus on the sensation of the breath moving in and out of your body.

Qigong for Reducing Work Stress

Qigong, an ancient Chinese practice that combines physical movements, breathing techniques, and meditation, has been shown to be effective in reducing stress in the workplace. Workplace stress is a major concern in many industries, with the potential to lead to burnout, decreased productivity, and negative impacts on physical and mental health. Qigong provides an accessible and practical way to manage work-related stress, with exercises that can be easily integrated into the workday.

One of the main benefits of Qigong for reducing work stress is its focus on relaxation and mindfulness. Many Qigong exercises are designed to release tension and promote relaxation in the body, allowing practitioners to enter a more peaceful and centered state of mind. This can be especially helpful for office workers who spend long periods sitting at a desk, often in positions that can lead to physical tension and discomfort.

One of the most popular Qigong exercises for reducing stress is the "Eight Brocades" or Ba Duan Jin. This set of eight exercises focuses on stretching and strengthening the body while promoting deep breathing and relaxation. The movements are designed to promote the flow of Qi or life force energy throughout the body, helping to release tension and improve overall well-being. The Eight Brocades can be practiced in a standing or seated position, making it a convenient choice for the office.

1. Another popular Qigong exercise for reducing stress is the "Five Animal Frolics" or Wu Qin Xi. This set of exercises is based on the movements of five animals: the tiger, deer, bear, monkey, and crane. Each animal

movement is designed to stretch and strengthen different parts of the body while promoting relaxation and mindfulness. The Five Animal Frolics can be practiced in a standing or seated position and can be adapted to suit different levels of fitness and mobility.

In addition to physical exercises, Qigong also includes breathing techniques and meditation practices that can be helpful in reducing work-related stress. One popular breathing technique is "Abdominal Breathing" or "Daoist Breathing," which involves deep breathing into the lower abdomen. This technique helps to calm the mind and relax the body, promoting a sense of well-being and inner peace.

Meditation is also an important component of Qigong, with many exercises designed to promote mindfulness and self-awareness. One popular Qigong meditation practice is the "Inner Smile" or Nei Wei, which involves imagining a smile spreading throughout the body, promoting feelings of joy and relaxation. Another popular meditation practice is "Standing Meditation" or Zhan Zhuang, which involves standing in a relaxed and balanced posture, focusing on the breath and the sensations in the body.

There are many benefits to integrating Qigong exercises into the workday for reducing stress. Studies have shown that regular practice of Qigong can help to reduce symptoms of anxiety and depression, improve overall physical health, and promote a sense of well-being and relaxation. In the workplace, Qigong can help to improve productivity, reduce absenteeism, and promote a positive and supportive work environment.

To get started with Qigong for reducing work stress, it can be helpful to find a qualified instructor or attend a class. Many workplaces now offer Qigong classes or wellness programs that include Qigong exercises. There are also many online resources and videos available that can provide guidance and instruction on Qigong exercises for reducing stress.

Qigong and Ergonomics

Qigong is a traditional Chinese exercise that promotes health and well-being. The practice of Qigong involves movements, postures, breathing techniques, and meditation. It has been found to be effective in reducing stress, improving physical function, and enhancing overall health. When combined with ergonomics, Qigong can be even more beneficial.

Ergonomics is the study of how people interact with their environment and is commonly applied in the workplace to promote health and safety. Ergonomics aims to design the environment to fit the person, rather than the person having to adapt to the environment. This can include adjusting furniture, equipment, and the work environment to prevent strain and injury.

Qigong and ergonomics can be combined to improve workplace wellness. Many office workers experience musculoskeletal pain and discomfort from sitting at a desk for extended periods. This can lead to back pain, neck pain, and other issues. Qigong exercises can help to alleviate this discomfort by improving circulation, reducing tension, and promoting relaxation.

One of the key principles of Qigong is proper alignment of the body. This involves maintaining a straight spine, relaxed shoulders, and a centered stance. When sitting at a desk, it is easy to slump forward and hunch over the keyboard, which can lead to strain on the back and neck. Practicing Qigong can help workers to maintain good posture and reduce the risk of musculoskeletal pain.

Qigong can also help to reduce stress and promote mental wellbeing. Many workers experience stress and anxiety in the workplace, which can lead to physical and mental health problems. Qigong breathing techniques and meditation can help to calm the mind and reduce stress levels. By practicing Qigong regularly, workers can improve their resilience to stress and promote their mental health.

In addition to promoting physical and mental wellbeing, Qigong can also improve productivity in the workplace. By reducing pain and discomfort, improving posture, and reducing stress, workers can perform their tasks more efficiently and effectively. Qigong can also help workers to maintain focus and concentration, which can improve their work output.

There are many Qigong exercises that can be practiced in the workplace. Some simple exercises include deep breathing, shoulder rolls, and spinal stretches. These exercises can be done while sitting at a desk and can be integrated into the workday. More complex exercises can also be practiced during breaks or outside of work hours.

It is important to note that Qigong should not replace ergonomics in the workplace. Ergonomic adjustments to the work environment, such as adjusting the height of the chair or monitor, should still be made to prevent strain and injury. Qigong exercises can be used in conjunction with ergonomics to promote overall workplace wellness.

Chapter Seventeen

Qigong Retreats and Workshops

Qigong, also known as chi kung, is a practice that involves movement, meditation, and breathing exercises that have been developed in China over thousands of years. Qigong has gained immense popularity across the world due to its numerous health benefits, and many people attend retreats and workshops to deepen their understanding of the practice. Below we will explore Qigong retreats and workshops, including what they entail and the benefits of attending one.

Qigong retreats and workshops provide participants with an immersive experience in the practice of Qigong. These retreats are typically held in natural and peaceful environments such as forests, mountains, or by the sea. The aim of these retreats is to create an environment that fosters relaxation, introspection, and personal growth.

At a Qigong retreat or workshop, participants will learn various Qigong exercises, meditation techniques, and breathing practices. The workshops are usually led by experienced Qigong instructors who have years of experience in the practice. Participants will have the opportunity to work closely with the instructors and receive personalized attention and guidance to deepen their practice.

In addition to learning the various Qigong practices, participants at Qigong retreats and workshops also benefit from being surrounded by a supportive community of like-minded individuals. The retreats provide a space where individuals can connect with others who are on a similar path of personal growth and self-discovery.

There are many benefits to attending a Qigong retreat or workshop. Firstly, these retreats provide a break from the hustle and bustle of daily life, allowing participants to disconnect from technology and connect with nature. The peaceful surroundings and immersion in the practice of Qigong can help reduce stress, anxiety, and promote relaxation.

Secondly, Qigong retreats and workshops provide an opportunity to deepen one's practice of Qigong. These immersive experiences allow participants to focus on their practice without the distractions of daily life. Participants can learn new techniques and refine their existing skills, with the guidance of experienced instructors.

Thirdly, attending a Qigong retreat or workshop can be a transformative experience. The combination of being surrounded by a supportive community, learning new techniques, and immersing oneself in the practice of Qigong can lead to personal growth and self-discovery. Many participants report feeling a renewed sense of purpose and clarity after attending a Qigong retreat.

Fourthly, Qigong retreats and workshops provide a space for participants to prioritize their health and well-being. The practice of Qigong has numerous health benefits, including reducing stress and anxiety, improving sleep quality, and enhancing overall physical health. By attending a Qigong retreat or workshop, participants can prioritize their health and well-being in a supportive and nurturing environment.

Finally, attending a Qigong retreat or workshop can be a fun and enjoyable experience. Many of these retreats are held in beautiful locations, providing an opportunity to explore new places and cultures while deepening one's Qigong practice.

Benefits of Attending a Qigong Retreat

Qigong is a form of traditional Chinese medicine that involves various breathing techniques, movements, and meditations. This practice has been gaining popularity worldwide due to its potential health benefits. Qigong can be practiced by anyone, regardless of age or physical ability, and can be done alone or in a group setting. One way to immerse yourself in the practice of Qigong is to attend a Qigong retreat.

A Qigong retreat is a structured program that offers participants the opportunity to deepen their Qigong practice in a supportive environment. These retreats can range in length from a weekend to several weeks and typically take place in peaceful and natural settings such as retreat centers, parks, or mountains. The focus of a Qigong retreat is to help participants relax, rejuvenate, and improve their health and well-being.

One of the main benefits of attending a Qigong retreat is the opportunity to learn from experienced Qigong teachers. These teachers are often experts in the practice and can provide guidance and instruction on the proper techniques and movements. They can also help tailor the practice to the individual needs of each participant, ensuring that everyone gets the most out of the retreat.

Another benefit of attending a Qigong retreat is the chance to connect with like-minded individuals. Qigong retreats attract people from all walks of life, and attendees often form lasting friendships and connections with others who share their interest in the practice. This sense of community can be empowering and inspiring, and can also provide a supportive network for continued practice and growth after the retreat is over.

In addition to learning from experienced teachers and connecting with others, attending a Qigong retreat can also provide an opportunity for self-reflection and personal growth. The peaceful and natural settings of many retreats can be a catalyst for introspection and self-awareness. Participants may find themselves better able to let go of stress and distractions, and instead focus on their inner selves and personal development.

The physical and mental health benefits of Qigong are well-documented, and attending a Qigong retreat can help amplify these benefits. Regular practice of Qigong has been shown to improve balance, flexibility, cardiovascular health, and immune function. It can also reduce stress, anxiety, and depression, and improve overall well-being. These benefits can be amplified by attending a retreat where participants can focus solely on their practice and immerse themselves in the healing environment.

Finally, attending a Qigong retreat can be a transformative experience. Many participants report feeling more centered, grounded, and energized after attending a retreat. They may also experience a greater sense of purpose or direction in their lives, as well as a renewed commitment to their health and well-being. This transformation can be a powerful motivator for continued practice and growth after the retreat is over.

Finding the Right Qigong Workshop

Qigong workshops and retreats offer participants the opportunity to deepen their practice, learn from experienced instructors, and connect with a community of like-minded individuals. However, with so many options available, finding the right workshop can be a daunting task. Below we will discuss some key factors to consider when choosing a Qigong workshop.

Firstly, it is important to consider the style of Qigong being taught at the workshop. Qigong has a variety of styles, each with its own unique movements and techniques. Some styles focus more on meditation and breathwork, while others emphasize physical movements and postures. It is important to choose a style that resonates with you and aligns with your personal goals and needs.

Secondly, consider the experience and credentials of the workshop instructor. Look for an instructor with a solid foundation in the specific style of Qigong being taught, as well as experience leading workshops and retreats. It can also be helpful to read reviews or speak with past participants to get a sense of the instructor's teaching style and ability to connect with students.

Another important factor to consider is the location and duration of the workshop. Choose a location that is easily accessible and conducive to your learning style, whether that be a remote nature retreat or an urban studio. The duration of the workshop can also vary greatly, from a single day to a week-long retreat. Consider your personal schedule and availability when choosing the duration of the workshop.

Additionally, it can be helpful to research the structure and content of the workshop. Some workshops may be focused on a specific aspect of Qigong practice, such as healing or martial arts, while others may offer a more comprehensive overview. Look for a workshop that aligns with your personal goals and needs, and consider the specific topics and techniques covered in the workshop.

Lastly, consider the cost of the workshop and any additional fees, such as accommodation or travel. While some workshops may be more expensive, they may also offer a higher level of instruction and more comprehensive programming. However, it is important to choose a workshop that is financially feasible for you and aligns with your personal budget.

Attending a Qigong workshop or retreat can offer a transformative and enriching experience for practitioners of all levels. By considering factors such as the style of Qigong being taught, the experience and credentials of the instructor, the location and duration of the workshop, the structure and content, and the cost, you can find a workshop that is the right fit for you.

Preparing for a Qigong Retreat Experience

Qigong retreats offer a unique opportunity to immerse oneself in the practice of qigong, surrounded by like-minded individuals in a peaceful and supportive environment. These retreats can range from weekend workshops to multi-week immersions in which participants can deepen their qigong practice, gain a greater understanding of the principles and philosophy of qigong, and experience profound personal growth.

If you are considering attending a qigong retreat, it is essential to prepare properly to make the most of your experience. Here are some tips to help you prepare for a qigong retreat experience:

Research the Retreat

First and foremost, it is essential to research the retreat before you commit to attending. Look for retreats that align with your interests, level of experience, and personal goals. Consider the length of the retreat, location, cost, accommodations, and the qualifications of the teachers. Additionally, read reviews from previous attendees to gain an understanding of the quality of the program and the experiences of those who have attended.

Prepare Mentally and Emotionally

Attending a qigong retreat can be a transformative experience, and it is essential to prepare yourself mentally and emotionally. Take some time to reflect on your reasons for attending the retreat and what you hope to gain from the experience. Be open to the possibility of personal growth and transformation, and approach the retreat with an open mind and heart.

Physical Preparation

Qigong retreats can be physically demanding, and it is essential to prepare your body for the experience. Engage in regular physical activity in the weeks leading up to the retreat, such as walking, yoga, or tai chi. Additionally, ensure that you are eating a healthy and balanced diet, drinking plenty of water, and getting enough rest.

Pack Appropriately

When packing for a qigong retreat, it is important to pack appropriately for the climate and environment. Check the weather forecast for the location of the retreat and pack accordingly. Additionally, bring comfortable clothing that allows for ease of movement, such as loose-fitting pants and shirts. Don't forget to pack a good pair of shoes for walking and hiking, as well as any necessary personal items such as medication, toiletries, and a water bottle.

Meditation and Breathwork

Meditation and breathwork are an integral part of qigong practice, and it is essential to familiarize yourself with these practices before attending a qigong retreat. Begin a regular meditation practice in the weeks leading up to the retreat, even if it is just a few minutes a day. Additionally, focus on deep, diaphragmatic breathing and explore various breathing techniques to gain a greater understanding of how breathwork can enhance your qigong practice.

Be Present

Finally, one of the most important things to remember when attending a qigong retreat is to be present in the moment. Disconnect from technology and the outside world as much as possible and allow yourself to fully immerse in the experience. Engage with your fellow retreat participants, ask questions, and participate fully in the retreat's activities. Remember that this is a unique opportunity to deepen your qigong practice, gain a greater understanding of the principles of qigong, and experience profound personal growth.

* 9 7 8 1 7 7 6 9 6 8 2 2 0 *

SD - #0206 - 070926 - C0 - 229/152/7 - PB - 9781776968220 - Matt Lamination